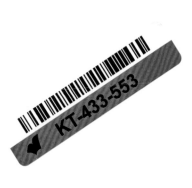

How to Write a Paper

Second edition

How to Write a Paper

Second edition

Edited by

George M Hall

Professor of Anaesthesia, University of London, and
Chairman of the Board of the
British Journal of Anaesthesia

First published in 1994
by the BMJ Publishing Group, BMA House, Tavistock Square,
London WC1H 9JR

First edition 1994
Reprinted 1994, 1995, 1996, 1997, 1998
Second edition 1998

British Library Cataloguing in Publication Data

A catalogue record for this book is available from the
British Library

ISBN 0-7279-1234-8

Typeset, printed, and bound in Great Britain by
Latimer Trend & Company Ltd, Plymouth

Contents

Contributors

R N Allan
Consultant Physician,
Gastroenterology Unit,
Queen Elizabeth Hospital,
Birmingham

Michael Doherty
Professor of Rheumatology,
Rheumatology Unit,
City Hospital,
Nottingham; Editor, *Annals of the Rheumatic Diseases*

G B Drummond
Senior Lecturer,
University Department of Anaesthetics,
Royal Infirmary,
Edinburgh;
Editorial team, *British Journal of Anaesthesia*

Michael J G Farthing
Professor of Gastroenterology,
Digestive Diseases Research Centre,
St Bartholomew's and the Royal
London School of Medicine and Dentistry,
London

Ian Forgacs
Consultant Physician,
Department of Gastroenterology,
King's College Hospital,
London

George M Hall
Professor of Anaesthesia,
University of London, and
Chairman of the Board of the *British Journal of Anaesthesia*

M J Halsey
Assistant Registrar,
Research and Commercial Services Office,
University of Oxford,
Oxford; Editorial Board Member,
British Journal of Anaesthesia and *Anaesthesia and Analgesia*

Richard Horton
Editor, *The Lancet*,
London

J S Lilleyman
Professor of Paediatric Oncology,
St Bartholomew's and the Royal
London School of Medicine and Dentistry,
London; Former Editor, *Journal of Clinical Pathology*

Maurice Long
Business Development,
BMJ Publishing Group,
London

John Norman
Professor,
Shackleton Department of Anaesthetics,
General Hospital,
Southampton; Former Postgraduate Editor,
British Journal of Anaesthesia

Norma Pearce
Technical Editor,
BMJ Publishing Group,
London

G Smith
Professor of Anaesthesia,
University of Leicester; former Editor, *British Journal of Anaesthesia*

Richard Smith
Editor, *British Medical Journal*

Alastair A Spence
Professor of Anaesthetics,
University of Edinburgh; former Editor,
British Journal of Anaesthesia

Stephen G Spiro
Professor of Respiratory Medicine/Clinical Director of Medicine,
University College London Hospitals

J A W Wildsmith
Professor of Anaesthesia,
Department of Anaesthesia,
Ninewells Hospital and Medical School,
Dundee; Editorial team, *British Journal of Anaesthesia;*
Associate Editor, *Regional Anaesthesia*

Alex Williamson
Publishing Director,
BMJ Publishing Group,
London

Preface to
second edition

The unexpected success of the first edition of this short book and the rapid progress in certain areas of publishing have necessitated a second edition. The original intention was that it would appeal primarily to authors for whom English was not their first language. However, sales in the United Kingdom show that it has met a local need. For the second edition it is a pleasure to welcome Professors Michael Farthing and Stephen Spiro, and Drs Richard Horton and Ian Forgacs as new contributors. Two additional chapters have been added: "Ethics of publication" and "Who should be an author?"

I am grateful to all authors for revising their chapters. In some instances few changes have been made but several authors have undertaken major revisions. I thank all contributors for the enthusiasm and commitment which they have brought to the project.

George M Hall
1998

1 Structure of a scientific paper

GEORGE M HALL

The research you have conducted is obviously of vital importance and must be read by the widest possible audience. It is probably safer to insult a colleague's spouse, family, and driving rather than the quality of his or her research. Fortunately, there are now so many medical journals that your chances of not having the work published somewhere are small. Nevertheless, the paper must be constructed in the approved manner and presented to the highest possible standards. There is no doubt that editors and assessors look adversely on scruffy manuscripts, regardless of the quality of the science. All manuscripts are constructed in a similar manner, although there are some notable exceptions such as the format used by *Nature*. These exceptions are unlikely to trouble you in the early stages of your research career.

The object of publishing a scientific paper is that you provide a document which contains sufficient information to enable readers to:

- assess the observations you made
- repeat the experiment if they wish
- determine whether the conclusions drawn are justified by the data.

The basic structure of a paper is summarised by the acronym IMRAD, which stands for:

Introduction	(What question was asked?)
Methods	(How was it studied?)
Results	(What was found?)
And	
Discussion	(What do the findings mean?)

The following four chapters deal with a specific section of a paper so sections will be described only in outline in this chapter.

Introduction

The introduction should be brief and must state clearly the question that you tried to answer in the study. To lead the reader to this point it is necessary to review briefly the relevant literature.

Many junior authors have difficulties in writing the introduction. The most common problem is the inability to state clearly what question was asked. This should not occur if the study was planned correctly. It is too late to rectify basic errors when attempting to write the paper. Nevertheless, some studies seem to develop a life of their own and the original objectives can easily be forgotten. I find it useful to ask collaborators from time to time what question we hope to answer. If I do not receive a short clear sentence as an answer, then alarm bells ring.

A review of the literature must not appear in the introduction. Only cite those references that are essential to justify your proposed study. Three citations from different groups are usually sufficient to convince most assessors that some fact is "well known" or "well recognised", particularly if the studies are from different countries.

Many research groups write the introduction to a paper before the work is started, but you must never ignore pertinent literature published during the conduct of the study. For example:

> It is well known that middle-aged male runners have diffuse brain damage [1,2,3], but whether this was present before running or arises as a result of repeated cerebral contusions during exercise has not been established. In the present study we examined cerebral function in a group of sedentary middle-aged men before and after a six month exercise programme. Cerebral function was assessed by . . .

Methods

This important part of the manuscript has become increasingly neglected and yet the methods section is the most common cause of absolute rejection of a paper. If the methods used to try to answer the question were inappropriate or flawed, then there is no salvation for the work. Chapter 3 contains useful advice about the design of the study and precision of measurement that should be considered when the work is planned, not after the work has been completed.

The main purposes of the methods section are to describe, and sometimes defend, the experimental design and to provide sufficient detail so that a competent worker can repeat the study. The latter is particularly important when you are deciding how much to include in the text. If standard methods of measurement are used then appropriate references are all that is required. In many instances "modifications" of published methods are used and it is these that cause difficulties for other workers. To ensure reproducible data, authors should:

- give complete details of any new methods used
- give the precision of the measurements undertaken
- use statistical analysis sensibly.

The use of statistics is not covered in this book. Input from a statistician should be sought at the planning stage of any study. Statisticians are invariably helpful and have contributed greatly to improving both the design and analysis of clinical investigations. They cannot be expected, however, to resurrect a badly designed study.

Results

The results section of a paper has two key features: there should be an overall description of the major findings of the study; and the data should be presented clearly and concisely.

It is not necessary to present every scrap of data that you have collected. There is a great temptation to give all the results, particularly if they were difficult to obtain, but this section should contain only relevant, representative data. The statistical analysis of the results must be appropriate. The easy availability of statistical software packages has not encouraged young research workers to understand the principles involved. The analysis presented must pass what is called in Chapter 4 the "Mark I Eyeball Test", sometimes known as the "BOT" (b . . . obvious test). An assessor is only able to estimate the validity of the statistical tests used, so if your analysis is complicated or unusual expect your paper to undergo appraisal by a statistician.

You must strive for clarity in the results section by avoiding unnecessary repetition of data in the text, figures, and tables. It is worth while stating briefly what you did *not* find, as this may save other workers in this area from undertaking unnecessary studies.

Discussion

The initial draft of the discussion is almost invariably too long. It is difficult not to write a long, detailed analysis of the literature that you know so well. However, a rough guide to the length of this section is that it should not be more than one third of the total length of the manuscript (Introduction + Methods + Results + Discussion). Ample scope often remains for further pruning.

Many beginners find this section of the paper difficult. It is possible to compose an adequate discussion around the points in the box.

Box 1.1 Writing the discussion

- Summarise the major findings
- Discuss possible problems with the methods used
- Compare your results with previous work
- Discuss the clinical and scientific (if any) implications of your findings
- Suggest further work
- Produce a succinct conclusion

Common errors include repetition of data already given in the results section, the belief that your methods were beyond criticism, and the preferential citing of previous work to suit your conclusions. Good assessors will seize upon such mistakes, so do not even contemplate trying to deceive them.

Although IMRAD describes the basic structure of a paper, there are other important parts of a manuscript. The title, summary (or abstract), and list of authors are described in Chapter 6. It is salutary to remember that many people will read the title of the paper and some will read the summary, but very few will read the complete text. The title and summary of the paper are of great importance for indexing and abstracting purposes, as well as enticements to persuade the reader to peruse the complete text. The use of appropriate references for a paper is described in Chapter 7; this is an area commonly full of mistakes. A golden rule is to list only relevant, published references and present them in a manner that is appropriate for the particular journal. The citation of large numbers of references is an indicator of insecurity, not of scholarship. An authoritative author knows the important references that are appropriate to the study.

Before you start the first draft of the manuscript, read carefully the "Instructions to authors" which every journal publishes and prepare the paper accordingly. Some journals give detailed instructions, often annually, and these can be a valuable way of learning some of the basic rules. It is a grave mistake to submit a paper in the style of another journal; this suggests that it has been rejected recently. At all stages of preparation of the paper, go back and check with the instructions to authors and make sure that your manuscript conforms. It seems very obvious, but if you wish to publish in the *European Annals of Andrology* do not write your paper to conform with the *Swedish Journal of Androgen Research*. Read and re-read the instructions to authors.

Variations on the IMRAD system are sometimes necessary in specialised circumstances, such as a letter to the editor (Chapter 8), an abstract for presentation at a scientific meeting (Chapter 9), or a case report (Chapter 10). Nevertheless, it is a fundamental system that is the basis of all scientific papers.

2 Introductions

RICHARD SMITH

Introductions should be short and arresting and tell the reader why you have undertaken the study. This first sentence tells you almost everything I have to say and you could stop here. If you were reading a newspaper, you probably would – and that is why journalists writing a news story will try to give the essence of their story in the first line. An alternative technique used by journalists and authors is to begin with a sentence so arresting that the reader will be hooked and likely to stay for the whole piece.

I may mislead by beginning with these journalistic devices, but I want to return to them: scientific writing can usefully borrow from journalism. But let me begin with writing introductions for scientific papers.

Before beginning, answer the basic questions

Before sitting down to write an introduction you must have answered the basic questions that apply to any piece of writing:

- What do I have to say?
- Is it worth saying?
- What is the right format for the message?
- What is the audience for the message?
- What is the right journal for the message?

If you are unclear about the answers to these questions then your piece of writing – no matter whether it's a news story, a poem, or a scientific paper – is unlikely to succeed. As editor of the *British Medical Journal*, every day I see papers where the authors have not answered these questions. Authors are often not clear about what they want to say. They start with some sort of idea and hope that the reader will have the wit to sort out what's important. The reader will not bother. Authors also regularly choose the wrong format – a scientific paper rather than a descriptive essay or a long paper rather than a short one. Not being clear about the audience is probably the commonest error and specialists regularly write for generalists in a way that is entirely inaccessible.

Another basic rule is to read the instructions to authors of the journal you are writing for. Too few authors do this, but there is little point in writing a 400 word introduction when the journal has a limit for the whole article of 600 words.

Tell readers why you have undertaken the study

The main job of the introduction is to tell readers why you have undertaken the study. If you set out to answer a question that really interested you, then you will have little difficulty. But if your main reason for undertaking the study was to have something to add to your curriculum vitae, it will show. The best questions may arise directly from clinical practice and, if that is the case, the introduction should say so:

> A patient was anaesthetised for an operation to repair his hernia and asked whether the fact that he used Ecstasy four nights a week would create difficulties. We were unable to find an answer in published medical reports and so designed a study to answer the question.

Or:

> Because of pressure to reduce night work for junior doctors we wondered if it would be safe to delay operating on patients with appendicitis until the morning after they were admitted.

If your audience is interested in the answer to these questions then they may well be tempted to read the paper and, if you have defined your audience and selected the right journal, they should be interested.

More commonly, you will be building on scientific work already published. It then becomes essential to make clear how your work adds importantly to what has gone before.

Clarify what your work adds

Editors will not want to publish – and readers will not want to read – studies that simply repeat what has been done several times before. Indeed, you should not be undertaking a study or writing a paper unless you are confident that it adds importantly to what has gone before. The introduction should not read:

> Several studies have shown that regular Ecstasy use creates anaesthetic difficulties,[1-7] and several others have shown that it does not.[8-14] We report two further patients, one of whom experienced problems and one of whom did not, and review the literature.

Rather it should read something like:

> Two previous studies have reported that regular Ecstasy use may give rise to respiratory problems during anaesthesia. These studies were small and uncontrolled, used only crude measurements of respiratory function, and did not follow up the patients. We report a larger, controlled study, with detailed measurements of respiratory function and two year follow up.

Usually, it is not so easy to make clear how your study is better than previous ones and this is where the temptation arises to give a detailed critique of everything that has ever gone before. You will be particularly tempted to do this because, if you are serious about your study, you will have spent hours in the library detecting and reading all the relevant literature. The very best introductions will include a systematic review of all the work that has gone before and a demonstration that new work is needed.

The move towards systematic reviews is one of the most important developments in science and scientific writing in the past 20 years.[1] We now understand that most reviews are highly selective in the evidence they adduce and often wrong in the conclusions they reach.[2] When undertaking a systematic review an author poses a clear question, gathers all relevant information (published in whatever language or unpublished), discards the scientifically weak material, synthesises the remaining information, and then draws a conclusion.

To undertake such a review is clearly a major task, but this ideally is what you should do before you begin a new study. You should then undertake the study only if the question cannot be answered and if your study will contribute importantly to producing an answer. You should include a brief account of the review in the introduction. Readers will then fully understand how your study fits with what has gone before and why it is important.

"In 1998 you should not worry that you cannot reach this high standard because the number of medical papers that have ever done so could probably be numbered on the fingers of one hand." I wrote the same sentence in the first edition of this book only with the year as 1994. I then wrote: "But by the end of the millennium brief accounts of such reviews will, I hope, be routine in introductions." I was – as always – wildly overoptimistic. Summaries of systematic reviews are still far from routine in introductions in scientific papers. Indeed, a paper presented at the Third International Congress on Peer Review in September 1997 showed that many randomised controlled trials published in the world's five major general medical journals failed to mention trials that had been done before on the same subject.

So my advice remains a counsel of perfection, but it's still good advice. Perhaps you can be somebody who moves the scientific paper forward rather than somebody who just reaches the minimum standard for publication.

Another important and relevant advance since the first edition is that scientific journals are beginning to have websites and to publish synergistically on paper and on the Web.[3] This at last opens up the possibility of simultaneously being able to satisfy the needs of the reader–researcher, who wants lots of detail and data, and the needs of the reader–practitioner, who wants a straightforward message. In the context of introductions, this means that a proper systematic review might be published on the Web while the paper version might include a short and simple summary.

Keep it short

You must resist the temptation to impress readers by summarising everything that has gone before. They will be bored, not impressed, and will probably never make it through your study. Your introduction should not read:

> Archaeologists have hypothesised that a primitive version of Ecstasy may have been widely used in ancient Egypt. Canisters found in tombs of the pharaohs ... Sociological evidence shows that Ecstasy is most commonly used by males aged 15 to 25 at parties held in aircraft hangars ... The respiratory problems associated with Ecstasy may arise at the alveolar–capillary interface. Aardvark hypothesised in 1926 that problems might arise at this interface because of ...

Nor should you write:

> Many studies have addressed the problem of Ecstasy and anaesthesia.[1–9]

With such a sentence you say almost nothing useful and you've promptly filled a whole page with references. You should choose references that are apposite, not simply to demonstrate that you've done a lot of reading.

It may often be difficult to make clear in a few words why your study is superior to previous ones, but you must convince editors and readers that it is better. Your introduction might read something like:

> Anaesthetists cannot be sure whether important complications may arise in patients who regularly use Ecstasy. Several case studies have described such problems.[1-4] Three cohort studies have been published, two of which found a high incidence of respiratory problem in regular Ecstasy users. One of these studies was uncontrolled[5] and in the other the patients were poorly matched for age and smoking.[6] The study that did not find any problems included only six regular Ecstasy users and the chance of an important effect being missed (a type II error) was high.[7] We have undertaken a study of 50 regular Ecstasy users with controls matched for age, smoking status, and alcohol consumption.

A more detailed critique of the other studies can be left for the discussion. Even then, you should not give an exhaustive account of what has gone before but should concentrate on the best studies that are closest to yours. You will also then be able to compare the strengths and weaknesses of your study with the other studies, something that would be wholly out of place in the introduction.

Make sure that you are aware of earlier studies

Editors know that it is easy to miss important earlier studies. Journals may publish studies in which authors proudly give the results of the first study on a problem, only for people to write in saying that they did an identical study 10 years ago. We have certainly had this experience several times at the *British Medical Journal* and we are always keen to see evidence that authors have made a determined effort to locate previous studies.

This search should obviously be undertaken before the study is begun, not when it is being written up. It is in nobody's interest to expend time and money exploring a question that has already been well answered. Before beginning a study, authors should seek the help of librarians in finding any earlier studies. Authors should also make personal contact with people who are experts in the subject and who may know of published studies that library searches do not find, unpublished studies, or studies currently under way. It's also a good idea to find the latest possible review on the subject and search the references and to look at the abstracts of meetings on the subject. We know that library searches often do not find relevant papers that have already been published, that many good studies remain unpublished (perhaps because they reach negative conclusions), and that studies take years to conduct and sometimes years to get into published reports.

Editors increasingly want to see evidence that authors have worked hard to make sure that they know of studies directly related to theirs. This is particularly important when editors' first reaction to a paper is "Surely we know this already". We regularly have this experience at the *British Medical Journal* and we then look especially hard to make sure that authors have put effort into finding what has gone before.

In a systematic review the search strategy clearly belongs in the methods section, but in an ordinary paper it belongs in the introduction, in as short a form as possible. Thus it might read:

> A Medline search using 15 different key phrases, personal contact with five experts in the subject, and a personal search of five recent conferences on closely related subjects produced no previous studies of whether grandmothers suck eggs.

Be sure your readers are convinced of the importance of your question, but don't overdo it

If you have selected the right audience and a good study then you should not have to work hard to convince your readers of the importance of the question you are answering. One common mistake is to start repeating material that is in all the textbooks and that your readers will know. Thus, in a paper on whether vitamin D will prevent osteoporosis you do not need to tell your readers what osteoporosis and vitamin D are. You might, however, want to give them a sense of the scale of the problem by giving prevalence figures for osteoporosis, data on hospital admissions related to osteoporosis, and figures on the cost to the nation of the problem.

Don't baffle your readers

Although you don't want to patronise and bore your readers by telling them things that they already know, you certainly don't want to baffle them by introducing, without explanation, material that is wholly unfamiliar. Nothing turns readers off faster than abbreviations that mean nothing or references to diseases, drugs, reports, places, or whatever that they do not know. This point simply emphasises the importance of knowing your audience.

Give the study's design but not the conclusion

This is a matter of choice, but I ask authors to give a one sentence description of their study at the end of the introduction. The last line might read:

> We therefore conducted a double blind randomised study with 10 year follow up to determine whether teetotallers drinking three glasses of whisky a week can reduce their chances of dying of coronary artery disease.

I don't like it, however, when the introduction also gives the final conclusion:

> Drinking three glasses of whisky a week does not reduce teetotallers' chances of dying of coronary artery disease.

Other editors may think differently.

Think about using journalistic tricks sparingly

The difficult part of writing is to get the structure right. Spinning sentences is much easier and editors can much more easily change sentences than structure. Most pieces of writing that fail do so because the structure is poor and that is why writing scientific articles is comparatively easy – the structure is given to you.

I have assumed in this chapter that you are writing a scientific paper. If you are writing something else you will have to think much harder about the introduction and about the structure of the whole piece. But even if you are writing a scientific paper you might make use of the devices that journalists use to hook their readers.

Tim Albert, a medical journalist, gives five possible openings in his excellent book on medical journalism:[4] telling an arresting story; describing a scene vividly; using a strong quotation; giving some intriguing facts; or making an opinionated and controversial pronouncement. He gives two examples from the health page of *The Independent*. Mike Hanscomb wrote:

> In many respects it is easier and less uncomfortable to have leukaemia than eczema . . .

This is an intriguing statement and readers will be interested to read on to see if the author can convince them that his statement contains some truth. Jeremy Laurance began a piece:

> This is a story of sex, fear, and money. It is about a new treatment for an embarrassing problem which could prove a money spinner in the new commercial National Health Service . . .

Sex, fear, and money are emotive to all of us and we may well want to know how a new treatment could make money for the health service rather than costing it money. My favourite beginning occurs in Anthony Burgess's novel *Earthly Powers*. The first sentence reads:

> It was the afternoon of my eighty-first birthday, and I was in bed with my catamite when Ali announced that the archbishop had come to see me.

This starts the book so powerfully that it might well carry us right through the next 400 or so pages. (I had to look up "catamite" too. It means "boy kept for homosexual purposes".)

To begin a paper in the *British Journal of Anaesthesia* with such a sentence would be to court rejection, ridicule, and disaster, but some of the techniques advocated by Tim Albert could be used. I suggest, however, staying away from opinionated statements and quotations in scientific papers, particularly if they come from Shakespeare, the Bible, or *Alice in Wonderland*.

Conclusion

To write an effective introduction you must know your audience, keep it short, tell readers why you have done the study and explain why it's important, convince them that it is better than what has gone before, and try as hard as you can to hook them in the first line.

1 Chalmers I. Improving the quality and dissemination of reviews of clinical research. In: Lock S, ed. *The future of medical journals*. London: BMJ Books, 1991:127–48.
2 Mulrow CD. The medical review article: state of the science. *Ann Intern Med* 1987;**104**:485–8.
3 Bero L, Delamothe T, Dixon A, *et al*. The electronic future: what might an online scientific paper look like in five years' time? *BMJ* 1997;**315**:1692–6.
4 Albert T. *Medical journalism: the writer's guide*. Oxford: Radcliffe, 1992.

3 Methods

G B DRUMMOND

The methods section should describe, in logical sequence, how your study was designed and carried out and how you analysed your data. This should be a simple task when the study is complete. However, if you leave writing the methods until this stage, you may only then recognise flaws in the design that you would have detected sooner if you had written this part in as much detail as possible *before* the study started. An experienced colleague could help by looking through this description to find weaknesses. The challenge of setting down what you intend to do is also a very useful exercise, far better than finding out after months of hard work that you should have used a different strategy, measured an additional variable, or anticipated and catered for a predictable requirement.

Testing hypotheses

When readers turn to the methods section, they are looking for more than details of the apparatus or assay that you used. They want to know exactly what hypothesis was tested: for example, that an intervention should result in a particular effect such as an increase in survival or improvement in outcome. This is tested by assuming that the null hypothesis is true. The observed results are used to assess how tenable this hypothesis can be, that is, the possibility that the intervention is without effect. The expression of how small this possibility (p value) has to be to disprove the null hypothesis should be stated clearly as the "mission statement" of the study. A study of two antibiotics might compare cure rate: the null hypothesis is that there is no difference, using cure as the outcome variable. A p value of less than 0.05 (out of a total probability of 1) implies that values less than this will make the null hypothesis untenable. Many papers merely say, adequately, "$p < 0.05$ was considered significant".

The other side of the coin of probability, often neglected, is the *power* of the study. Readers should not be encouraged to believe that, if the null hypothesis has survived your attempts to destroy its credibility, there is probably no difference between the groups. This negative outcome may be either true or false: you have not shown that your methods are sufficient to test the null hypothesis. First, a true difference may be present, but it might only be a small one. Second, there may be a difference but the measurements might be variable enough to swamp the effect. In both cases, there is a small "signal-to-noise" ratio. Your methods should, if possible, give an estimate of the power of the study to detect what you are looking for, so that the reader can assess the possibility of a false negative result. This is the β error. The value you choose may depend on factors such as the precision of the answer needed and the practical consequences of an incorrect conclusion, but it is often taken as 0.2, which implies a *power* of 0.8 to avoid a false negative result. In practice, the power of a study depends on the size of the effect, the variability of the data, and the number of observations.

Always state clearly the *a priori* hypotheses, if only to be sure that you collect appropriate and relevant data and do the correct statistical tests.

Statistics

Give the exact tests used to analyse the data statistically, with an appropriate reference if the test is not well known. If a computer was used, then give the type of computer, the software, and the software version. The choice of statistical test depends on the type of data. It may not be clear before the data are collected whether parametric tests can be used, in which case the *a priori* tests should be non-parametric.

Design

The study design can often be described in a few well chosen words, particularly if it is a description of a layout of the groups or events. The groups may be *independent,* allocated to different treatments, and the design is often *parallel,* each group receiving a different treatment, with both groups being entered at the same time. In this case comparisons will be between groups. Subjects receiving different treatments may be *paired,* to reduce the effects of confounding variables such as weight or sex. The effects of a treatment on each subject may be assessed before and after; such comparisons are *within subject.* The simplest study design is a *randomised parallel design* with a comparison of outcome between groups.

Box 3.1   What to include in the methods section

How the study was designed:

- Keep the description brief
- Say how randomisation was done
- Use names to identify parts of a study sequence

How the study was carried out:

- Describe how the subjects were recruited and chosen
- Give reasons for excluding subjects
- Consider mentioning ethical features
- Give accurate details of materials used
- Give exact drug dosages
- Give the exact form of treatment and accessible details of unusual apparatus

How the data were analysed:

- Use a *p* value to disprove the null hypothesis
- Give an estimate of the power of the study (the likelihood of a false negative – the β error)
- Give the exact tests used for statistical analysis (chosen a *priori*)

Always state clearly how randomisation was done, since this is a crucial part of many clinical trials. The method used should be stated explicitly in this section. Specific aspects such as blocked randomisation (to obtain roughly similar group sizes) and stratification (to obtain a balance of confounding variables such as age or sex in each group) must be described. Authors often choose wrong forms of randomisation such as alternate cases, the unit number, date of birth, and so on. Correct methods involve the use of random number tables or closed envelope methods. In a study that involves blind assessment you may need to describe how the assessor was kept unaware of the treatment allocation.

A diagram may be helpful if the design of the study is complex or a complicated sequence of interventions is carried out. You can help readers by using explicit names for the separate parts of a study sequence so that they can follow the results; names or even initials are preferable to indicate groups or events rather than calling these events 3, 4, 5, and so on.

Subjects and materials

Readers want to know how the subjects were recruited and chosen. Healthy, non-pregnant (probably male) volunteers may not reflect the clinical circumstances of many occasions when a drug is used. Try to give an indication of what disease states have been excluded and how these diseases were defined and diagnosed. What medication leads to exclusion from the study? Alcohol and tobacco use can alter drug responses and it is tempting to exclude subjects who drink and smoke, but the results are less applicable to clinical practice. A list of the inclusion and exclusion criteria set out in the ethics application form may be helpful.

Although most journals indicate that ethical approval is a prerequisite for acceptance, some ethical features of study design may need to be mentioned. For example, you may need to describe some of the practical problems of obtaining informed consent or of obtaining a satisfactory comparative treatment.

In a laboratory study, details such as the source and strain of animals, bacteria, or other biological material, or the raw materials used are necessary to allow comparisons to be made with other studies and so that others could repeat the study you have described. Give exact drug dosages (generic name, chemical formula if not well known, and proprietary preparation used if relevant) and how you prepared solutions, with their precise concentrations.

The exact form of treatment used has to be described in a way to allow replication. If the methods, devices, or techniques are widely known or can be looked up in a standard text – the random zero sphygmomanometer or a Vitalograph spirometer, for example – then further information is unnecessary. Similarly, widely used apparatus such as the Fleisch pneumotachograph does not require further description, but less well known apparatus should be described by giving the name, type, and manufacturer.

Methods that are likely to be uncommon or unique should be described fully or an adequate reference to the method should be provided. Readers object if a reference of this sort is only to an abstract or a limited description in a previous paper. If in doubt, provide details and indicate how the methods were validated.

The apparatus used must be described in sufficient detail to allow the reader to be confident of the results reported. Is the apparatus appropriate, sensitive enough, specific in its measurement, reproducible, and accurate? Each aspect may need to be considered separately. For example, bathroom scales may fulfil all these criteria when used to estimate human body weight, as long as they have been checked and calibrated recently. On the other hand an inadequate chemical assay may be non-specific because it responds to other substances, gives different results when the same sample is tested twice (poor reproducibility), and gives results that are consistently different from the value expected when tested against a standard substance (poor accuracy). The method may not detect low concentrations (insufficient sensitivity).

The methods used to standardise, calibrate, and assess the linearity and frequency response of the measuring devices used may need to be described. Such characteristics should be given when high fidelity measurements are reported. Do not merely repeat the manufacturer's data for accuracy of a piece of apparatus, particularly if it is crucial to the study: the standard used for a calibration must be stated and the results of the calibration quoted. If analogue to digital conversion is done in computerised analysis, an indication of the sampling rate and accuracy of sampling procedure is necessary. Similar considerations of adequate description apply to other methods of assessment and follow up, such as questionnaires, which should be validated.

Box 3.2   A good methods section can answer these questions

- Does the text describe what question was being asked, what was being tested, and how trustworthy the measurements of the variable under consideration would be?
- Were these trustworthy measurements recorded, analysed, and interpreted correctly?
- Would a suitably qualified reader be able to repeat the experiment in the same way?

Recommended reading

Begg C, Cho M, Eastwood S, *et al.* Improving the quality of reporting of randomized controlled trials: the CONSORT statement. *JAMA* 1996;**276**: 637–9.

Eger EI. A template for writing a scientific paper. *Anesth Analg* 1990;**70**: 91–6.

4 The results

JOHN NORMAN

The results section provides the answers to the questions you, as the author, pose in the introduction. The answers will most likely be the ones you were expecting. Sometimes they will not and you may refute your original ideas. Occasionally something unexpected comes up and you need to report it. Serendipity has a part to play.

What you must avoid is what any reader, editor, or assessor dreads: "The results are presented in Tables I to V and in the figures." This does not guide the readers into discovering what you want them to find but actively encourages them to find things you do not think important. You must lead your readers into following your thoughts, usually by using a mixture of text, tables, and illustrations.

First, you will need to describe the subjects of your studies in enough detail for the readers to assess how normal or abnormal they were. Readers need to compare these with their own subjects. You might have given these details in the methods section but it is becoming common for this information to appear in the results. Avoid calling the characteristics of the subjects the "demographics". According to the *Shorter Oxford Dictionary* demography is the branch of anthropology studying the statistics of births, deaths, and diseases.

The next section presents the answers. Start with some text. In general, the readers will follow the text as though it were telling a story, so start at the beginning and go on logically to the end. Use the tables to present the meat of the results and to establish the statistical validity of your conclusions. Illustrations should be used for emphasis of the important points. The eye and the brain are good at picking up a message from pictures; working through a mass of numbers is much harder. Remember that both the tables and the illustrations should be capable of standing alone. There must be sufficient information associated with them for the reader not to have to refer back to the text. Think that a reader might want to copy them to illustrate the next public lecture – with due acknowledgement!

Always use words; add the tables and illustrations when necessary.

The words

Tell the story of how you arrived at the answers. Establish initially how normal or abnormal your groups were and how comparable they were. Even with a random allocation into groups, it is necessary to confirm that they are equivalent. One in 20 such allocations will produce statistically significantly different groups. Many journals will be printing 20 papers in each issue – yours could be the unlucky one. If your groups do differ in this way, you will have to comment and state, in the discussion, how those differences affect the interpretation of your results.

Having established the baseline, the story can be developed in a number of ways. You might want to show an example of a typical response and use an illustration. The reader will assume that your typical response is in fact your most dramatic one but we are all human. Then summarise, in the text, the answers to your main questions. Give an indication of the size of any effects and their statistical significance. In the discussion, you will deal with the practical as opposed to the statistical significance. If your results do not support your original ideas or even refute them, you still need to describe them. Take comfort from Sir Karl Popper's advocacy of learning by refuting hypotheses. Such results should make you, and your readers, think again and come up with better ideas.

You will almost certainly come up with some unexpected results. The final part of the section should illustrate these, state their statistical significance, and lead to a development in the discussion section of what they mean.

The statistics

Many papers suffer because the statistics are presented badly. Many statistical tests can be used, some familiar and others more esoteric. Your planning of the study will include the decision as to which tests to use. You will not have taken the results to your local statistician to see what can be made of them. That wastes everyone's time. But even with the right tests it is not easy to condense the results into the space available. But, please try!

In general, do not give results to a greater degree of accuracy than that of the measurement. If you can only measure cardiac output with an accuracy of $\pm 10\%$ do not quote values for individual results to three significant figures. The convention for describing means does allow you to use one more significant figure than for the individual results. The same applies to standard deviations and errors and confidence limits. Take care that any statistically significant changes you want to emphasise are greater than the errors of your measurements. Take extra care with calculated values: the errors of the original measurements add up alarmingly.

If you are using proportions of groups with various attributes, do not use percentages unless the groups contain more than 100 subjects.

Usually, there will be insufficient space in the text or the tables for you to present all your data. You will need to condense the material but not to an extent where the reader (and assessor) cannot follow you. Suppose for a group of subjects you have measured some characteristic – perhaps the weight of each patient. Rather than give each individual result you can condense the findings. You need to give the number in the group, the range of the results, some measure of the central tendency, and some measure of the spread. Spread is often given by the probability of where the mean lies (for example, the standard error or the confidence limits for the mean) but you might want a measure of the spread of values of the whole group (for example, the standard deviation or the coefficient of variation). Choose the set of values according to the answer you need for your original question. If the distributions are not normal then use either a transformation to make them appear normal or other descriptors such as the median and its confidence interval and the quartiles. The goal is to give as much information as possible in the smallest space.

Often, the results you wish to show involve a time series with repeated measurements made over the course of a treatment. You wish to emphasise where significant changes are seen. The table of results is likely to show these as a series of mean values plus the measures of spread. Your statistical analysis will almost certainly be a variant of an analysis of variance. You ought to include the table for that analysis showing the sources of variance, the associated degrees of freedom and the F values. This happens rarely. Without it, the assessor of the paper will resort to the cruder t test to check your conclusions. That can lead to a delay in having the paper accepted. With these more complex tests there is a case for including with your paper an extra table of all the results marked as being for "editorial and assessor's use only". These individuals can then repeat your tests (or use their own). You can also offer to let readers have full copies of the data should they so desire. But remember that, if your statistical tests are esoteric and not reported in full, the assessor is likely to use the crude "Mark I Eyeball" test. Be prepared then for a lengthy discussion before publication.

There are similar problems if you are looking at associations between variables. The statistical significance needs to be brought out to emphasise how much of the association can be attributed to the dependency of one variable on another and how much is due to chance. Beware of extrapolation. Beware of confusing association with causation. There is the story of the high degree of correlation between the salaries of Baptist ministers in New York with the price of rum in Havana!

But these matters should have been cleared at the planning stage. Statistical presentation is always a problem – so much information and so little space. Present enough for the intelligent reader to believe what you are saying.

The tables

You will be able to show a vast amount of data in the tables. In general, do not use the tables you prepared to accompany a talk. Those tables should have been designed for rapid assimilation of key points only by the audience. (You would never use a larger format than five columns by four rows at a talk, would you?)

The key is to make each table deal with a specific problem. Use the first to describe the general characteristics of your subjects. Use the remaining ones to give details of the answers. If you want the reader to look at changes, remember that most readers in the Western World work naturally from left to right, not from top to bottom. So present the results in columns where the changes run from the left-most column. Often, it helps to present results as percentage changes from the initial value. If you do this, include

Table 4.1 Cardiovascular response to intubation

Event	Heart rate	Systolic BP	Diastolic BP	Cardiac output
Premedication	75 ± 12	135 ± 14	87 ± 10	4.408 ± 0.714
Induction	72 ± 5	115 ± 12	71 ± 13	3.728 ± 1.135
Intubation	95 ± 10	179 ± 19	110 ± 32	4.693 ± 1.948
Anaesthesia	82 ± 8	130 ± 14	78 ± 12	4.296 ± 1.547

This is a poor table. The title does not explain what is intubated. Most of the grid lines are superfluous. The columns have no indication of the units used. The results for cardiac output are almost certainly showing more significant figures than can be justified. The symbol $\pm$ is not defined (standard error or deviation?) and there is no indication of the number of subjects studied. Further, the changes occur by going down, not across, the page. There is no indication of any statistically significant change.

Table 4.2 Cardiovascular changes during establishment of anaesthesia

	Premedication	Post-induction	Post-intubation	Anaesthesia
Heart rate beats/min	75 ± 12 (62–104)	72 ± 5 (54–94)	$95 \pm 10^*$ (72–124)	82 ± 8 (65–104)
Systolic BP mm Hg	135 ± 14 (105–155)	115 ± 12 (87–152)	$179 \pm 19^*$ (125–219)	130 ± 14 (94–155)
Diastolic BP mm Hg	87 ± 10 (67–107)	71 ± 13 (53–92)	$110 \pm 32^*$ (92–145)	78 ± 12 (55–102)
Cardiac output l/min	4.4 ± 0.7 (3.2–6.0)	3.7 ± 1.1 (2.4–5.2)	4.7 ± 1.9 (2.9–6.8)	4.3 ± 1.5 (2.4–6.5)

The values for 10 subjects are the means, standard deviations, and ranges for the variables measured after premedication, after induction of anaesthesia, immediately after tracheal intubation, and five minutes after establishing anaesthesia. Statistically significant differences ($p<0.05$) from the initial values are shown by *. The significant changes were the increases in heart rate and systolic and diastolic blood pressures following tracheal intubation. This table is set out in a more standard form and includes much more information. It could be improved further by adding a secondary table showing the results of a two way analysis of variance.

an initial column of actual figures as well (see the sample tables, Tables 4.1 and 4.2).

Make your presentation match the statistical analysis that you have done. It is annoying to have results in the tables as means and standard deviations when a non-parametric test is being used. Ensure that you use enough, but not too many significant figures. If your numbers have been processed through a computer, remember that they will work to many more figures than you need. Make the numbers match the measurements.

Tables 4.1 and 4.2 illustrate what is often submitted and how the information can be made to look much better.

One final point. Use the "Instructions to authors" for the journal or a recent copy to ensure that the format of your tables matches those that are published. Not only does it flatter the editor by making him think you read the journal but it saves time in setting up the material in print. Few papers use vertical lines in their published papers: many word processing packages include them automatically.

The illustrations

Good illustrations will get your message across clearly. The mind takes in pictorial information much more quickly than written text. Good illustrations will display the data and lead the reader to think about the substance of the answers you provide. They can reveal data at several levels. Tufte's books (see the Recommended reading list) are excellent guides as to what can and should be done. Only some key points can be given here. Talk to your local medical artists but remember that what may please them visually may hide your messages. Also, remember that illustrations have to go through a number of processes before appearing in print. Each process will lose some detail so make the quality of your originals as high as you can. Properly drawn material is better than laser which, in turn, is better than an ink-jet, which is much better than a dot-matrix printer. But not all illustrations come from the personal computer.

The illustrations you made for the talk to the learned society are often useless for a journal. They will have been made for rapid assimilation by the audience while you were talking to them. In print, illustrations can contain more detail but also appear much smaller. Many journals will print your illustrations on a half-page width (in one column) to save paper. Most will be in portrait form, rather than the landscape format usually used with talks. (This has a slight advantage in that it will emphasise any significant changes seen in the results plotted on the ordinate.)

Next, many journals do not routinely print illustrations in colour. This is changing but unless colour is vital (as with pictures of patients or pathology) you might be asked to pay for the extra costs of colour. Further, the glorious colours used in many computer graphics programs will need extensive revision to make good black-and-white pictures.

Photographs and micrographs

Photographs must include measures to protect the anonymity of any patient and micrographs need measures of scale. Both need professional production.

Reproduction of records

If you have a good trace of an experimental result, use it. Traces of the arterial pressure changes accompanying tracheal intubation, with and without your therapeutic intervention, will make the points rapidly. But take care with the traces. Ensure that both the time and the pressure axes are calibrated. Talk to the photographers to ensure that the trace is highly visible. If there is a background grid, ensure that it does not predominate. Many heat sensitive papers produce a blue trace on a red grid. When photographed, the blue gets lost and the red grid predominates. There are papers that will give a black trace on a green paper. There are also papers with no grid which can be useful as long as you supply the calibration marks. Some photographic paper, such as that which is sensitive to ultraviolet light, is excellent for fast events but it is difficult to prepare a black-and-white print from it and it needs protection from sunlight. Talk to your photographer.

Graphics

Most illustrations are drawings made to bring out the highlights of the paper. Remember the value of good diagrams that summarise the protocol of your investigation. But the others will be used to bring out the highlights of the results presented in the tables and text.

Computer graphics offer an enormous variety of pictures. Three dimensional representations of bar graphs, pie charts, and surfaces are almost irresistible. But use these only as a last resort to bring out a point. The eye and brain assess three dimensional bars as volumes, not lengths. Tufte's books illustrate some classic mistakes based on this. Make sure that the printer's ink goes on data and

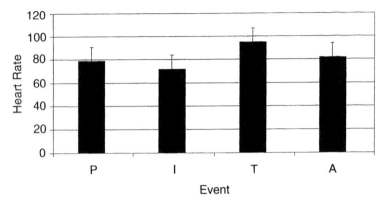

Figure 4.1   Heart rate measurements after premedication (P), induction of anaesthesia (I), tracheal intubation (T), and five minutes later (A). The data are taken from Table 4.1 and show the mean values as the heights of the bars plus the T bar showing one standard deviation. (This figure uses too much ink; the ordinate does not give the units and the horizontal grid is probably not needed. The figure needs either the title or the legend for the ordinate: heart rate does not need repeating. There are no marks to show the significant faster rate after tracheal intubation.)

not on what Tufte calls "chartjunk". The best guide will be the illustrations presented in the current issues of the journal. Most editors and publishers are keen to present quality – even to the extent of employing professional artists to redraw pictures to a common house style. If you can present them with the material already in that format, then your acceptance rate will rise.

Figures 4.1 and 4.2 use the heart rate data from the tables; Figure 4.1 uses a lot of ink but shows little information while Figure 4.2 reduces the amount of ink and shows much more data.

Finally, for both illustrations and tables, remember that they must stand alone. Your readers must be able to interpret them without recourse to the text of the results or, ideally, to other figures and tables. Each one needs an appropriate legend. Abbreviations must be defined, as must each symbol. If you use ± state whether it is for the standard deviation or the error. (You don't need to use it at all – you can define the number as a deviation or error without the symbol.) Draw the reader's attention to any highlights and to any marks showing where statistically significant events occur. Follow the "Instructions to authors" and, should you have the misfortune to have the paper refused by the

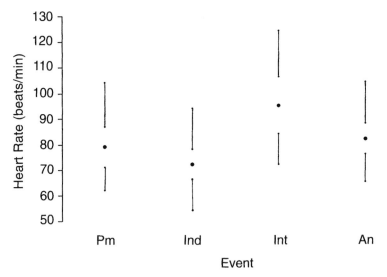

Figure 4.2   Heart rate measurements after premedication (Pm), induction of anaesthesia (Ind), tracheal intubation (Int), and after stabilisation of anaesthesia (An). The data are from 10 patients; the central dot represents the mean values and the surrounding bars identify the range (outer end) and 95% confidence limits of the mean (inner ends). The rate after tracheal intubation is statistically significantly (p<0.05) greater than at the other times. (This may be a more appealing picture: it gives more information and the eye easily follows the flow of the changes seen.)

first journal, check the instructions for the second one. Editors may not look kindly on material which is obviously in the format for another journal.

Conclusion

The results section is the easiest one to write. The introduction has defined the questions and the methods the ways of getting the answers. You should have thought in the design stage how the results will be presented and you will have planned the appropriate mixture of text, tables, and figures. Indeed, apart from filling in the data in the tables and placing the dots in the figures, you could almost write the results as you start the work. You shouldn't – if only because you will meet some surprises on the way. Remember that the text should tell the story, that the tables will summarise the evidence, and that the illustrations will show the highlights. Keep it all straightforward and at all times – *remember the reader.*

Recommended reading

O'Connor M. *Writing successfully in science*. London: Chapman & Hall, 1991. (An excellent guide to the whole business.)

Tufte ER. *The visual display of quantitative information*. Cheshire, CT: Graphics Press, 1983. (This is a *tour de force* showing what is too often done and what can be done.)

Tufte ER. *Visual explanations*. Cheshire, CT: Graphics Press, 1997. (How to use graphics to get your point across. Anaesthetists and epidemiologists will love the comparison of John Snow's work on cholera in 1854 and the problems facing the *Challenger* space shuttle in 1986.)

5 Discussion

ALASTAIR A SPENCE

The discussion section, no less than the other parts of the paper, is an exercise in logic and discipline. It should state the main findings of the study. It should highlight any aspect of the methods that is less than you aimed for (assuming, of course, that this is not a significant confounding factor). You should note previously published findings in the same area of endeavour and, if necessary, try to explain any inconsistency between your work and that of others. Finally, what are the implications of your findings for practice or for future research, or both? These aspects are discussed with the help of imagined examples.

The main findings

In this study patients who received cyclizine 10 mg intravenously at the end of anaesthesia were half as likely to complain of nausea in the ensuing six hours as those who received intravenous saline (17% v 36%). There was no obvious adverse effect associated with receiving cyclizine.

The two sentences encapsulate the main conclusion of the study without repeating the data, which must be confined to the results section. It is a useful discipline to try to describe the major findings in a sentence or two before starting to write the manuscript. Among other benefits, this will provide an excellent start to the discussion.

Previous work

In many cases it is likely that perusal of previous publications has been the stimulus to methods for the present paper. New technology may have become available, allowing more precise

31

assessment. In a previous publication or subsequently, flaws in the experimental plan may have occurred. The present paper offers a new look at the problem. Sometimes it is appropriate to note a previous study in the introduction to a paper. That is not a reason for excluding a reference in the discussion section, but the repeat reference should add something substantial to the narrative.

In 1971 Black and White reported no improvement in the incidence of postoperative pulmonary complications associated with the use of a rebreathing tube. Their assessment, however, was based on X-ray changes and oral temperature, which are obviously less specific than the scanning methods we have used. On the other hand, the difference between treatment groups is very similar to that reported by Pink and Blue (1991) in patients recovering from open cholecystectomy: the rebreathing tube had a sparing effect on FRC reduction (21% v 38% in controls).

Inexperienced authors often write a long and detailed critique about every paper ever written on the subject. This merely indicates the thoroughness of the literature search; it is necessary to confine your attention to the major players. There are often only a few reputable research groups active in a particular area and their previous work must be discussed. The judgment of what to put in and what to omit may be difficult; senior colleagues can help with this decision.

Discussion of method

A recognised difficulty in studies of this type is variability in recall of events in the reproductive history (Walker and Jones, 1987). We believe that limiting the period studied to the previous two years is likely to have minimised the source of error.

It is most unlikely that the methods you used in the study were perfect, so you should present a brief appraisal in the discussion. This is particularly important if the design of the study was unusual; you may need to defend vigorously this aspect of the investigation. Hopefully, you will have improved on the methods used previously to examine the topic – this is therefore an opportunity to show your work in a good light and even gently chide rivals on the deficits of their work.

What it means for practice

Our findings confirm the value of prophylactic heparin in preventing pelvic vein thrombosis in patients undergoing abdominal hysterectomy. In our large series of 780 patients not a single significant complication of extradural local anaesthetic injection could be found. As a result, the use of heparin in this setting has become part of our hospital practice guidelines.

If your findings may alter clinical practice, then this should be discussed. Similarly, if the study was non-clinical, then any basic scientific implications must be mentioned. Most authors are unlikely to make a major breakthrough and it is probable that you have only added another small piece to a large scientific jigsaw. Even so, it is important to state how our scientific understanding has progressed, albeit very little, as a result of your work.

The need for further study

Although we are much encouraged by the apparent brain protection associated with infusion of omphagon in our rat model, further study of the longer term effects on the brain will be needed before the use of the drug in humans is justified. Also, the risk of hepatotoxicity must be defined in view of the occasional finding of hepatocellular injury in these experiments.

A contributor to the *British Journal of Anaesthesia*'s guide has observed wryly that the prudent investigator might wish to be well established in the further study before urging the idea on the world at large! This assumes, however, that you will continue in this area of work. If this is unlikely, then you may wish to claim precedence in the discussion for suggesting the next steps in the investigation of the problem.

Some authors like to finish the discussion with a succinct résumé of the major findings. There is a risk of repetition, however, as the same information is likely to have been reported in the abstract (or summary), in the results section, and at the beginning of the discussion. The editor may then simply delete this part of the

33

manuscript in the interests of brevity and clarity. There is a trend away from completing the manuscript in this traditional manner.

Acknowledgments

This part of the paper can be an Achilles' heel, for a variety of reasons. The source of research funding should always be acknowledged. Failure to do so is likely to constitute a violation of the conditions under which an award has been given. Even if that is not obviously the case, it is still important to acknowledge who provided financial support. Within the published literature as a whole there are an extraordinary number of studies, which must have consumed resources that someone has paid for, which do not mention this. Another related matter is that journal editors (and readers) increasingly need to know if a commercially interested body has provided support. Under some circumstances this might raise the question of whether the author is involved in a "conflict of interest".

Acknowledge anyone (for example, colleague, nurse, technician) whose work, as distinct from attitude of mind, enabled the study to proceed. Anyone who has contributed to the originality of the work should be considered as a co-author. The best way to ensure that this aspect has been handled properly is to make certain that any individuals involved at that level have been consulted about the manuscript for publication or are aware of who appears as a co-author and who appears in the acknowledgments section. At the same time the acknowledgments section should not be seen as a catch-all for anyone you wish to flatter or do not wish to offend. The appearance of an individual's name in the acknowledgments might to some extent implicate that person if there is any controversy about the work once it is published. Again, you are covered if there is appropriate consultation before submission to an editor.

By all means recognise secretaries, wives or husbands, lovers, and parents, but not in the manuscript. There have been occasions when editors or their assistants may have put more into the final drafting of a manuscript than the authors, but it is never appropriate to mention their contribution in your acknowledgments!

34

Aims of discussion

- To state the main findings
- To highlight any shortcomings of the methods
- To compare the results with other published findings
- To discuss the implications of the findings.

6 Titles, abstracts, and authors

J S LILLEYMAN

Face facts. Richard Asher was right. Medical journals are dull. Their intrinsic dullness is the product of several influences including (in no particular order) literary inability, fear of frivolity, editorial timidity, and peer pressure perpetuating custom and practice. And, I suppose, the need for structure and precision in scientific writing. But there is dull and there is very dull. Many published papers fall squarely into the latter category, which is inexcusable.

People write scientific papers for a variety of reasons. Their ranks are greatly swelled by those who feel it is obligatory for their career but have no relish (or aptitude) for the task, and also those who do so purely to satisfy research funding bodies rather than because they have something new or exciting to tell the world. We probably have to thank authors like this (and the pressures that drive them) for the ridiculous and growing number of biomedical journals – supply following demand to ensure that most manuscripts, however trivial, boring, or badly written, will eventually appear somewhere. As Asher says, "Every dull dog has his day".[1]

Since most medical papers describe studies of underwhelming importance, to make them very dull to boot is a double crime. Every effort should be made to avoid the compounding felony and a good way to start is to pay particular attention to titles and abstracts. These components form the packaging and essence of an article and, thanks to the efficiency of electronic literature searching and abstracting, are all that most people will ever see or read. With that sobering thought, let us consider each in turn.

Titles

Whether your article eventually appears in an obscure specialist publication with 98 subscribers (97 of whom are members of the editorial board) or a journal with a household name, a six figure worldwide circulation and a press conference following every issue depends, of course, on what it is about and how novel or important it is. But it also depends to a greater extent than might be realised on how well written and interestingly presented it is and the title is an important beginning.

Too few authors realise how much the time spent on this vital part of their creation will be rewarded. When a manuscript arrives on an editor's desk, the title is the first thing that will be seen. It can immediately prejudice the way the paper is handled – whether it is scanned immediately, put to one side, or handed to someone else. When a paper is published, it is the title that the reader sees first in the contents list and the casual browser might or might not be seduced into turning to the appropriate page. More importantly, the committed reader, a worker in the same field, might miss a relevant paper on "first pass" if the title is elliptical or obscure.

To be fair, there is not much advice about titles contained in most "Instructions to authors". The guidelines of the International Committee of Medical Journal Editors (Vancouver Group)[2] do not dwell on the topic beyond indicating that titles should be "concise and informative" and few journals comment specifically on the matter when describing their house style. One exception is the *New England Journal of Medicine*, which states that "titles should be concise and descriptive (not declarative)". This useful tip means that authors should resist the challenge of trying to condense the whole of their paper into the title, results, conclusions, and all – an exercise attempted surprisingly often.

So how should a title be constructed?

Above all else, it should convey, in easily understood terms, what the paper is about. It should also be as short as possible and it should excite rather than stifle interest.

1. Indicate subject matter

When describing what the paper is about, do just that. Do not say why it was written, what the findings were, or what conclusions were drawn. Let the reader know the topic of the report, not its detailed contents.

Exactly how a title should be worded depends to some extent on the journal to which the article is being submitted. The target readership may be (a) laity, (b) medical workers from outside your own specialty, (c) professionals within your own broad specialty, or (d) the cognoscenti within your own superspecialty. You may reflect this in the use or avoidance of technical words but, generally, a golden rule is the simpler the better. Trendy jargon should always be avoided. Apart from obscuring meaning, such language often has a short shelf life and dates your publication as effectively as flared jeans.

So, take an imaginary manuscript with the clumsy draft title:

> An epidemiological geographically based study of the quantity and effects of ionising radiation received by male employees of a nuclear reprocessing plant and nearby male residents working elsewhere in the same vicinity shows an increased risk of childhood leukaemia in the children of the nuclear workers only.

Remove the conclusion and stick to saying what it is about in simple language. Try instead:

> An epidemiological study of radiation received by male employees of a nuclear reprocessing plant and other residents in the vicinity and its relation to the incidence of childhood leukaemia.

But that is still far too long. It needs to be much shorter and more interesting.

2. Be brief

When Polonius lengthily explained to Gertrude about brevity being the soul of wit, he might usefully have added that it is also vital for successful communication in writing. Short titles tend to be more arresting. They also take up less space, are usually clearer, and are inevitably preferred by editors. When you think that the title you have arrived at is as short and pithy as possible, it is worthwhile seeing how many more words can be squeezed out of it without loss of meaning. It is also quite enjoyable as an intellectual exercise. Definite articles can usually be dispensed with (though that is a matter of style) and excessive adjectives or "noun salads" (a string of nouns masquerading as adjectives to form clumsy phrases like "reader pain threshold increase") can usually be ruthlessly pruned.

Revisit the leukaemia paper and now try:

Radiation to residents near a nuclear reprocessing plant and its relation to childhood leukaemia: an epidemiological study.

3. Be interesting

Finally, do not be afraid of attempting to provoke interest. As Asher put it, an author should try to make the title "allure as well as inform",[1] but be careful never to stray into the world of sensationalism. You are not indulging in the art form of writing headlines and "Leukaemia shock from nuclear waste dump" should be left to the tabloid professionals. Our epidemiology paper already has an arresting title, because the subject matter is politically sensitive as well as clinically important, but if we want to ensure that it has maximum impact for a general readership we might go as far as:

Nuclear reprocessing, radiation exposure, and childhood leukaemia: an epidemiological study.

This title still confines itself to conveying what the paper is about and is not misleading. It contains all the key words to help electronic retrieval to be achieved reliably. It is easy to understand, catches the eye, and provokes curiosity. The reader will now have to proceed at least as far as the abstract or summary to learn more. If that happens, the title will have served its purpose well.

Box 6.1   Guidelines for producing a good title

- The simpler the title, the better
- Consider the target readership
- Be brief – short titles are clearer and more arresting
- House style determines whether definite articles are left in
- Avoid excessive adjectives and noun strings
- Do not be sensationalist

Abstracts

Whether you call them abstracts or summaries, in this context the words mean the same. Both refer to a brief résumé of the chief points of a larger work.

After the title, the abstract is the second most read part (frequently the only other part read) of a paper and so is likely to be the basis on which the work is judged by uncritical readers. It is also the first part of a paper that an editor reads carefully and it may provoke the choice of referees.

Like the title, the abstract will reward time spent on it and should be short, intelligible, informative, and interesting. It should be a digest of the whole paper and contain its essence. It should stand alone and will then be helpful to those who, through electronic abstracting services, have access only to the summary and not the whole paper. There will be many such users. There will also be library readers of the whole paper who, for reasons of economy, may copy only the abstract to remind them of the contents. In short, there is every reason to spend a great deal of effort on getting an abstract as near perfect as possible and making it the most highly polished part of the paper.

Despite this, abstracts are often poorly constructed, meandering, and uninformative. Vital bits are left out or the reader is left hanging at the end as the authors weakly finish by saying that "the findings are discussed". Not much use if the main paper is not readily available and an annoyance that further effort is necessary even if it is. Frustrated editors of some journals have got so weary of trying to lick indifferent summaries into shape that they now insist that they be formally structured with labelled headings to make sure that the right bits go in and nothing gets left out.

So what should an abstract contain? It should consist of four basic parts, which can vary individually in length. These should describe succinctly:

- why what was done was done
- what was done
- what was found
- what was concluded.

The permissible length may be defined by the journal in question, but 200 words is a good average target that should be exceeded only in exceptional circumstances. The Vancouver Group suggests a maximum of 150 words for unstructured abstracts and 250 for fully structured formats.

1. A worked example

Consider each section of the abstract in turn and write it as a separate paragraph. *Why what was done was done* should contain one or two sentences to orientate the reader and indicate the reason for the study.

Snibbo is a novel compound for the treatment of road rage. A randomised double-blind placebo-controlled trial was carried out to assess its effectiveness.

What was done should briefly describe the methods used.

All white van drivers stopped by police on the M25 were invited to participate. Daily Snibbo (2 mg/kg) was compared with placebo. Participants were assessed at 0, one and four weeks by a standardised outside lane crawler test and their IQ adjusted apoplexy scores recorded.

What was found should include a synopsis of the results, including the size of the study groups and all basic figures.

One hundred volunteers were recruited: 48 received Snibbo and 52 placebo. There was no difference in the apoplexy scores at 0 and one week, but at four weeks those in the Snibbo group had a range of scores of 2–40 (median 22) compared with 17–82 (median 47) in the control group, showing a difference in median score of 25 (95% confidence interval 15–45; $p<0.01$).

What can be concluded records what can be learnt from the paper and should make clear its message to the world.

For the relief of road rage in those particularly at risk, Snibbo appears to be more effective than placebo, but only after it has been taken for more than one week.

2. Structuring an abstract

The *New England Journal of Medicine* would structure the above 160 word abstract by the same four paragraphs and head them Background, Methods, Results, and Conclusions. Just to be different, *The Lancet* would call them Background, Methods, Findings, and Interpretation. The *British Medical Journal*'s abstract structure is slightly more detailed and fussy. As well as asking for sections called Objectives, Results, and Conclusions, where appropriate it splits the "what was done" section into Design, Setting, Subjects, and Main Outcome Measures. But the principle is the same and other journals that use formal structured abstracts all follow a similar basic four-part template.

3. What to leave out

As well as making sure that the right things go into an abstract, it is helpful to be clear about what can be left out. There is no need for a flowery introduction which will be repeated in the appropriate section of the main paper and there is no need to describe the patients studied in detail, listing each and every exclusion. Methods can nearly always be left to the body of the text. Results should give adequate details of the main findings (including basic grouped figures, together with statistical confidence intervals and p values) but not what might be called epiphenomena, and conclusions should be clear and uncluttered without discussion drifting about "on the other hand".

4. Try reading it aloud

When finished, see if the text of the abstract flows by reading it aloud to a colleague unfamiliar with the work. This final test will highlight any remaining ambiguities or obscurities and will enable the final gloss to be applied. The process takes time. Remember, text that is easy to read is hard to write.

5. Key words

The Vancouver Group guidelines also suggest that up to 10 key words or phrases to assist indexers should be given at the end of abstracts. These should be based on the medical subject headings (MeSH) of *Index Medicus*, using categories in which you might search for such an article if you were doing a literature trawl yourself. If suitable MeSH terms are not available others can be used. For the above worked example, appropriate key words might include: "Road rage, Snibbo" (and incidentally, a suitable title for the paper might be "Snibbo for road rage: a randomised trial").

Box 6.2   Guidelines for producing a good abstract

- The abstract should contain the essence of the whole paper and should stand alone
- It should consist of four basic parts:

  why the study was done
  what was done
  what was found
  what was concluded

- Stick to a maximum of 150 words for an unstructured abstract and 250 for a structured one
- Be clear and concise and avoid unnecessary detail

Authorship

When considering the question of who should co-author a paper, the Vancouver Group is quite vociferous and restrictive.[2] It says that all authors should have made "substantial contributions" to (a) the concept and design of an experiment or analysis and interpretation of data; (b) drafting the article or revising it critically for important intellectual content; and (c) final approval of the version to be published: all three, not just one. General supervision of the research group or just participation in data collection or simply raising the funds for the project are not considered sufficient.

The Vancouver Group guidelines also suggest that, where large collaborative trials are concerned, the key people responsible for the article should be specified, with other contributors being listed separately in an acknowledgment.

All this has been the case for a few years, but there are recent signs that yet more restrictions are looming and some influential editors, provoked mostly by fear of fraud, want to change the traditional concept of authorship altogether. Rennie *et al*, in an outspoken article in the *Journal of the American Medical Association*, recently suggested that the concept of "authors" should evolve to that of "contributors" where it is explicitly stated in a list what role the various individuals played in preparing an article.[3] This,

43

it is claimed, will increase accountability and enhance the integrity of publications. It will certainly put paid to "gift authorship" and sticking the boss on the end of the list of every paper to keep him happy.

The Lancet and the British Medical Journal agree and both are now pursuing the notion of "contributorship" in an exploratory way.[45] Perhaps the mood is best summed up in The Lancet's current instructions:

> An author must have made significant contributions to the design *and* execution *and* analysis *and* writing up of the study, and he or she must share responsibility for what is published. We now ask authors to specify their individual contributions and we publish this information.

Some revisionist editors also want each paper to have at least one identified guarantor to carry the can for the whole work. They point out that presently there are too many instances of fraudulent research where nobody accepts responsibility.

The same motive drives virtually all editors to insist that all authors should sign a submission letter or a note of agreement to include them as authors. Some journals also require a declaration of participation in the study and qualification to be included as an author. If authors are scattered around the world, collecting autographs can take some time, so it is worth while doing this before the final version of the manuscript is ready to post. And ask the journal editor to return the co-authors' signatures if he rejects the article.

It is in the interest of authors (or contributors) to keep their numbers small if they like to see their names in reference lists or indexing and abstracting services. The ideal number is one or two: then both names are always quoted. With three or more, those not in pole position run an increasing risk of being consigned to *et al.* With more than six, those ranked seven or more may appear in print only in the original article.

So ask yourself quietly who qualifies as a masthead author. Keep the numbers down. Reflect whether Dr Morbid, who did some special histological stains on your case of Snibbo's disease, really qualifies to be a co-author or whether he was just doing his job and could be satisfied with a courteous acknowledgment as a footnote. The same might apply to Dr Neutron who carried out some extracurricular postmortem radiology. Remember that researchers or secretaries who type references into databases or

44

manuscripts love short author lists and detest the task of transcribing endless names.

They also love short titles, which brings us back to the beginning.

Box 6.3   Care for your readers, your editors, and yourself

Remember the following points:

- Provide short and interesting titles
- Painstakingly construct concise, readable, and informative abstracts
- Share the credit with as few people as possible and ensure that all co-authors really contributed

---

1 Asher R. *A sense of Asher: a new miscellany.* London: British Medical Association, 1984.
2 International Committee of Medical Journal Editors. Uniform requirements for manuscripts submitted to biomedical journals. *N Engl J Med* 1997;**336**:309–15.
3 Rennie D, Yank V, Emanuel L. When authorship fails. A proposal to make contributors accountable. *JAMA* 1997;**278**:579–85.
4 Smith R. Authorship is dying: long live contributorship. *BMJ* 1997;**315**:696.
5 Horton R. The signature of responsibility. *Lancet* 1997;**350**:5–6.

7 References

M J HALSEY

This chapter outlines the techniques for finding the appropriate references for a paper and subsequently presenting them correctly in the manuscript to be submitted for publication. One of the characteristics and strengths of all scientific research is that each investigation has as its foundation the work of predecessors in the field. Thus, knowledge of the published work is critical to the success and soundness of the study, as well as to the credibility of the paper.

Most people will already be aware of some of the publications on their topic. The practical questions are whether they have the key references; whether the references they propose to include in the paper are the right balance between being comprehensive and being relevant; and finally whether there are any new current references about which they ought to be aware.

Initial literature search

It is a cliché to bemoan the expansion of the medical literature, but the important aspect to remember is that it is all organised and systematically indexed. If you understand the basic systems it is relatively easy to gain an entry into the published work. The most widely used index system is *Index Medicus*, an index to periodical articles in the medical sciences covered by the (American) National Library of Medicine. This index is produced in monthly issues which are subsequently combined to produce a cumulative index for the year. The associated computer bibliographic database is Medline. Both indexes are international in scope; approximately 75% of the citations are published in English. More than 3700 journals are indexed and every article is classified by subject and author. The full text is not provided but approximately half the citations include the original abstract.

Classification by subject

Classification by subject is far more sophisticated than simply recording the authors and the title of the article. When an article is indexed for *Index Medicus* or Medline, the indexer at the National Library of Medicine assigns several (on average 10) single or multiterm terms for the most specific topics covered in the article. These medical subject headings (MeSH) are used to cover the central aspects of each article, as well as other significant information discussed in the article. On the other hand, ideas only mentioned in passing will not be indexed. The obvious advantage of this system is that it does not rely on the accuracy and completeness of the title or key words chosen by the original authors.

It is important to understand the ways in which these MeSH terms are structured. In general, the terms chosen for the index are as specific as possible. If the researcher searches the literature using a more general term, articles indexed under narrower subterms will not be found. This problem can be overcome in the printed version of *Index Medicus* by first consulting the list of MeSH terms and choosing the most appropriate one for a particular search. In the computer form of the index, Medline, there is a facility for "exploding" a term – that is, the system searches for the selected term plus all its narrower, more specific terms. With this technique you can find information that may not be indexed to the selected term but, because it is indexed to a narrower term, is pertinent to your topic.

It is also possible to limit the numbers of articles found by including a subheading that describes a specific aspect of the topic (for example, Adverse Effects, Diagnosis, or Pharmacokinetics). If you "explode" a single term, the subheadings are applied to each narrower term as well as to the term itself.

Limitations of the system

There are some limitations to the system which should be remembered. First, it is important to recognise that some key terms may have synonyms and variants as well as English or American spelling; these aspects can usually be overcome by use of the thesaurus facility. Second, it should be noted that acronyms are not usually indexed. For example, those searching for articles on

AIDS would retrieve articles on financial aids, etc but not acquired immune deficiency syndrome (which requires the full and specific spelling). Third, if you are searching back into the literature it must be remembered that there are historical changes in the index terms and even in the journals covered by the system; what may be a suitable search pattern for the current year is not necessarily going to reveal the appropriate articles from 1990. This is particularly true for pharmacological topics for which there was a major indexing change in 1996.

A general suggestion for checking the adequacy of the search strategy is to be aware of at least a couple of articles that should be retrieved and to check that they do show up. Alternatively, it is possible to check the MeSH headings used for the known articles and then apply these as part of the wider search.

Search systems

The computer based systems subdivide into those that operate online or via PCs or CD-ROMs: online search services include Medline, Dialog, PaperChase, and BRS. PC-based systems include Current Contents on diskette and Reference Update. The CD-ROM systems include Compact Cambridge and SilverPlatter.

The great advantage of a number of these systems (such as SilverPlatter) is that, in addition to the title, author, and MeSH terms, the abstract is also available. This enables the researcher to decide quickly if the particular article is relevant or only peripheral to the specific aspect of the topic under consideration. Inevitably such systems are not cheap and have been possible only because of the increased storage capacity provided, for example, by CD-ROMs. However, more medical libraries now have one or other of the systems available and this approach to literature searching is so much more efficient than manual alternatives.

Alternative indexes

Although *Index Medicus*, with Medline, has become the most widely used index system in medical research, it should not be forgotten that there are other indexes that serve specific needs.

Excerpta Medica (EMBASE), a major pharmacological and biomedical literature database, is subdivided into clinical specialties and has the advantage of providing a printed abstract (sometimes the authors' and sometimes prepared by a compiler who is an expert in the field). The subjects are subdivided into specific headings and provide a means of keeping up with a specific field of interest within a discipline. In general, the journals indexed are confined to clinical medicine and this should be borne in mind when reviewing a specific topic.

Biological Abstracts (abstracts and indexes of life sciences information) is an example of one of the other indexes which, in this case, concentrates on experimental medicine and the biological sciences. Another example is *Chemical Abstracts*, which dates from 1907 and was one of the original abstracting indexes.

Science Citation Index (bibliographic references from over 4400 journals in the fields of natural, physical, and biomedical science and technology) is a system that lists where a particular paper has been cited. It is very useful if a key reference is known and you want to know who has subsequently written on that topic. It is particularly appropriate when the terminology has not yet been included in the MeSH headings of *Index Medicus* and so the more conventional approaches to literature searching are not very efficient. One of its limitations is that it is based on only the first author of the article.

Five years' cumulative indexes – many specialist journals produce cumulative indexes of articles that they have published. This is a reasonable method of initiating a search into the literature, but it is important to know the index terms and subheadings used by any particular journal. Some specialties have standardised their index systems within the discipline, but there are inevitably some idiosyncrasies.

Box 7.1   List of printed indexes

- *Index Medicus*
- *Excerpta Medica*
- *Biological Abstracts*, *Chemical Abstracts* (both single year and five year collective index)
- *Science Citation Index*
- Journals' cumulative indexes

Box 7.2   List of computer databases

There are well over 700 in addition to Medline; examples of the larger ones include:

- Biosis – biology, including clinical and experimental medicine, immunology, pharmacology, biophysics, and biochemistry
- EMBASE (*Excerpta Medica*) – excludes nursing, veterinary medicine, and dentistry, but is particularly strong on drug-related literature
- Health – non-clinical, administration
- IPA – drug development
- Toxline   –   toxicology,   including   teratogens,   mutagens, carcinogens, pollutants, and pesticides; adverse drug reactions
- Zoological record – the world's most comprehensive index to zoological literature

---

Continuing literature awareness

There is a strong negative correlation between time since graduation and currency of knowledge. This may or may not be true for a particular individual, but all would acknowledge that it requires a conscious effort to keep up to date. This activity goes far beyond reading relevant publications and attending meetings. It is vital that articles can be remembered, that the citations are accurate, and, most important, that the previous work is quoted accurately. Several approaches help in this process.

Regularly reading one or more specialist journals should provide a significant yield of high quality articles directly relevant to your own interests and clinical practice. Many members of departments also meet in one of the many forms of "circulation club" which keep people abreast of a wider field within their discipline.

Review articles now form over 5% of the total scientific literature. Those appearing in specialist journals are usually written by accepted authorities in the field. They are not necessarily current because of the inevitable delays in the publication process, but this can be easily checked from the dates in the reference list. Some reviews (such as *Physiological and Pharmacological Reviews*) are not only written by accepted authorities but are also peer reviewed before acceptance for publication. This means that they are a carefully considered assessment of the current position in the field and can be regarded as milestones in the literature. Another type is the *Annual Review* series (of medicine, pharmacology, or physiology) or the *Recent Advances* series (in anaesthesia, etc). Some reviews are not necessarily as authoritative as others and the fact that a contribution is labelled as a review should not be taken as a seal of academic approval. There has been a proliferation of this type of derivative literature. Those who write reviews know that they are incredibly popular for reprint requests. Finally, it should be noted that there are now reviews of reviews and *Index Medicus* provides a special bibliography of medical reviews.

Conference proceedings have proved to be a useful source of current material. These are now indexed separately under the title *Proceedings in Print*. It should not be forgotten that often it is the conference itself that provides the peer review and as such the abstracts or precirculated papers may not be as authoritative as they appear. Theses are more carefully considered and are an underutilised source of current thinking in a particular field. The difficulty is access, but this has been helped by the publication of *The Index of Theses accepted for Higher Degrees* and *Dissertation Abstracts International*. The electronic version is ISTP (*Index to Scientific and Technical Proceedings*).

Current Contents provides simple lists of the contents pages of journals and is now available in weekly booklet or PC disk format. Some commercial companies provide these on a limited scale for journals in a particular discipline as a complementary service to the profession. The whole approach has become less cumbersome with the arrival of computer searching programs. These are based on the words in the titles and, as with Medline, combining a series of specific title words in a search pattern can be very effective in identifying key articles.

New computer systems are being developed all the time. Two examples are TEAL (The Electronic Anesthesia Library) and SIGLE (System for Information on Grey Literature). Grey literature is best described as not being available through normal channels and includes conference papers, technical and research reports, and doctoral dissertations.

Storage of references

Once you have acquired and read the relevant papers carefully, it is vital to make a note of the important information in them and to store the references so that they can be retrieved easily.

The traditional method of doing this is on record cards, but it should be noted that if you are going to be doing serious research for, say, three years you could easily accumulate over 1000 references and a manual system quickly becomes very unwieldly. It is for this reason that people use a computer storage and retrieval system.

There are now several personal reference management systems for use on PCs which are designed to record article citations and to help in the generation of bibliographies for papers. The literature references are entered either by using the keyboard or by linking to one of the search services. It is possible to enter notes or text of any length for each article (subject, of course, to your computer's storage capacity, which is surprisingly finite in this context). Once the references are entered, you can retrieve them by almost anything you can remember about them (author, keyword, title word or phrase, note, etc).

A major virtue of these programs is that they can generate bibliographies formatted in virtually any journal style and can incorporate the appropriate reference citations into a manuscript. It is not a just a question of making life easier. Using a computer generated reference section does ensure that the original references need be checked only at the time of entry, and the subsequent generation of drafts and revisions does not result in inaccuracies creeping into the pristine reference section.

A leading computer system in this area is Reference Manager. It was first developed in 1972 and many quirks have since been ironed out. It has the advantage that the program and a copy of the main database can be installed on as many computers as you wish. The only restriction is that the same database must be copied to each computer. Anyone purchasing for the first time should enquire about what and when will be the next update version and what will be its advantages.

Producing the reference section in a paper

Except for review articles, long lists of references are usually inappropriate. Restrict references to those that have a direct bearing on the work described. As a guide, it is rarely necessary to cite more than 40 works for the longest of papers. In general, cite only references to books listed in *Books in Print* or to articles published in journals indexed by *Index Medicus*.

There are two major methods of referring to the bibliographic material: the Vancouver system, which is becoming widely preferred,[1] and the Harvard system, which is retained by a few journals. Even if you know which system is used by the particular journal to which you wish to submit a paper, check the specific guide to contributors as well, because there are still many minor variations in the layout.

Don't regard the reference section of the paper as a minor chore to be left to the last moment or to the most junior author (or the secretary typing the paper). Submission of references that are inappropriate, inaccurate, or in the wrong format may appear to the inexperienced author to be only a technical issue, but to an editor it may be sufficient reason for returning the paper for retyping before even considering it. If it gets past the editorial office it is not unknown for assessors to recognise that the references are in the style of another journal and to conclude that the paper has already been rejected for publication at least once and to scrutinise the whole article more harshly.

Word processors enable reference lists to be corrected and amended, but the fact that a reference looks right is dangerously deceptive. There is a tried and tested way of finally checking the reference list: photocopy the first page of every reference cited; at the same time, make sure that this page includes all the details commonly needed in reference lists whatever the preferred format (for example, last page numbers, book publisher's name, and location). Keep these first pages with the hard copy of the evolving manuscript and use them to check directly both the final submitted version and the proof copy.

Box 7.3   Guidelines for producing a useful reference list

- Restrict the list to those references with a direct bearing on the work described
- For references to journal articles cite only references to journals listed in *Index Medicus*
- Check the house style on whether the Vancouver or Harvard system is used
- Check the "Instructions to authors" and make sure that you have included all the necessary details for each reference

The Vancouver system

References are numbered consecutively in the order in which they are first mentioned in the text. References in text, tables, and legends are identified by arabic numbers appearing in the text either in brackets (usually specified as square, but not by all journals) or as superscripts. The alternative variation on this, used for some review articles in journals otherwise conforming to the Vancouver system, is for the references to be arranged alphabetically in the reference list and numbered accordingly in both list and text.

Sometimes authors consider it essential to cite the names of authors of a study in the text (in addition to the identifying number). Here the convention is to cite only up to three names (Adams, Smith and Jones [24] have shown . . .). If there are more than three names it is better to use a phrase such as "Birt and colleagues [25]" or "Hall and co-workers [26]". The expression "*et al*" is not encouraged by most editors. Sometimes people use an informal reference to previous work (Nunn's study or Mushin's work) but in this case the paragraph must always contain the reference cited formally as well; this is usually at the end of the specific sentence.

The Harvard system

In this system the order of references at the end of the paper is strictly alphabetical, regardless of chronology. The style of citations varies slightly from journal to journal. In the text, references should be made by giving in parentheses the name of the author and the year of publication – for example, (Hall, 1988) – except where the author's name is part of the sentence – for example, "Hall (1988) showed that . . .". Where several references are given together they should be listed in chronological order and separated by semicolons. When a paper written by two authors is quoted, both names are given; if there are more than two authors all the names should be given the first time the reference is cited, but after that it is sufficient to give the first name only, adding *et al*. When two citations have the same author(s) and the same year of publication, alphabetical annotation is used – for example, (Nunn, 1991a) and (Nunn, 1991b). The order of alphabetically annotated citations should ideally be chronological within the year, but this is the counsel of perfection.

Guidelines common to both systems

Text references to "unpublished observations" or "personal communications" should not be included in the final list of references. "Unpublished observations" include information from manuscripts submitted but not yet accepted for publication; don't try to slip in another piece of work by including it in the reference list as "submitted for publication". If the other work is critically important to the present paper, wait until the former has been accepted for publication before submitting the present manuscript. "Personal communications" should be cited in the text as: [Brown AB, personal communication]. The authors have responsibility for ensuring that the exact wording of references to unpublished work is both seen and approved by the person concerned.

Papers that have been submitted and accepted for publication should be included in the list, the phrase "in press" replacing volume and page number. Authors should be prepared to give the volume and page number at the time of proof correction.

Format for the reference list

The list of references at the conclusion of the paper begins on a new sheet of paper. The easiest way of ensuring that you have the right format for this part is to look both at the journal's "Instructions to authors" and at a couple of reference lists in current papers in the same journal. If in doubt the usual convention is as follows.

Journal article – Surname and initials of all authors (not *et al*, however many authors), full title of paper, full title of journal (with capitalisation of both nouns and adjectives), year of publication, volume number (not issue number unless it is a supplement), first and last pages of article. Some parts of journals have letters following or preceding the page numbers (for example, P (for Proceedings), A (for Abstract), S (for Supplement)). If such designation letters are used they should always be included in the reference citation of the pages.

Book or monograph – Surname and initials of author(s), full title of book (usually underlined), number of edition, town of publication, publisher, year of publication. In general, it is desirable to be as specific as possible in a book reference so add specific pages to the quotation if they are relevant but don't make the citation too complex or repetitive.

Chapter in a multiauthor book – Chapter author, initials, chapter title, book authors (or editors), and initials, book title, town of publication, publisher, year of publication, first and last pages.

Proceedings of conferences – Only include these if the proceedings have been published in an *Index Medicus* journal or in a recognised book. In the former case use the journal format (with a designation letter if included); in the latter case use the book chapter format (with the designation "Proceedings of . . ." if it appears in the book title).

Conclusion

The importance of the reference section of a paper is sometimes underestimated by inexperienced authors. In fact, it is critical to the credibility of the paper. In 1985 an analysis of the quotations and references in medical journals revealed serious deficiencies.[2] It was discovered that 20% of the references appearing in the *British Medical Journal* were misquoted, with half of these misquotations being seriously misleading. In the *British Journal of Surgery* as many as 46% of all citations were wrong, with 39% of these errors being major (that is, the article could not be located).

Since that time editors, assessors, and reviewers have been determined to improve the situation. Inaccurate quotations and citations are displeasing for the original author and misleading for the reader and mean that untruths become "accepted fact". Current authors should be aware that, if their reference sections are not of the highest standard, it is they who will be castigated by future generations of researchers attempting to search the literature.

1 International Committee of Medical Journal Editors. Uniform requirements for manuscripts submitted to biomedical journals. *BMJ* 1991;**302**:338–41.
2 De Lacey G, Record C, Wade J. How accurate are quotations and references in medical journals? *BMJ* 1985;**291**:884–6.

8 How to write a letter

MICHAEL DOHERTY

General considerations

When wishing to submit a letter to a journal, first consider the following basic questions:

- What is the purpose of your letter?
- Is a letter format appropriate for this particular journal?
- Does what you want to say justify a communication?

The purpose of a letter varies between journals (Box 8.1). Most letters are comments in response to a previous publication, though brief communications that do not justify a full report are sometimes appropriate as letters. It is always wise to read the "Instructions for authors" and to examine the correspondence section of recent issues of the journal to gain a feel for the style and scope of successful (that is, published!) letters. Because the amount of

---

Box 8.1 The purpose of a letter

Usual:

- Comment against or in favour of a previous publication
- Communication of case report(s)
- Concise communication of clinical or investigative data

Less common:

- General medical or political comment (for example, "guild issues")
- Comment concerning the nature or format of the journal
- Advertisement of interest to collaborate or gain access to patients or study material

---

information provided in a letter is necessarily limited, there is rarely justification for more than three authors.

Always question whether the information you wish to convey truly justifies publication – minor comments or observations are unlikely to be accepted. If the purpose and content of your communication seem appropriate as a letter, two other major considerations are its length and the style of presentation. With respect to length, always be brief. All journal editors like concise communications. They would rather publish 10 short letters on 10 different topics than two lengthy ones on only two. Think how you react as a reader – messages are always more effective if put briefly. Some journals impose firm restrictions on length, number of references, and use of accompanying tables or figures. This will be in the "Instructions to authors" but, even if it is not overtly stated, all editors favour a Raymond Chandler over a Charles Dickens. For example, compare the following two extracts.

Sir,

I feel I must put pen to paper with respect to the recent communication by Dr Peter Jones and colleagues in your August issue[1] to draw the attention of your readers to possible misinterpretation of the data presented. Although these excellent workers have a proven track record in the field of complement activation (not only in rheumatoid arthritis but in other inflammatory diseases as well), in this present study they appear to have omitted to properly control for varying degrees of inflammation in the knee joints of the patients that they aspirated – not only those with rheumatoid arthritis but also those with osteoarthritis. Such inflammation of the knee joint could have been assessed either by local examination and scoring for features such as temperature increase, effusion, synovial thickening, anterior joint line tenderness, duration of early morning stiffness, and duration of inactivity stiffness, with addition of the different scores to a single numerical value (that is, the system devised and tested by Robin Cooke and colleagues in Alberta[2]) and/or by simultaneous measurement and comparison to levels of other markers of inflammation, for example, the synovial fluid total white cell and differential (particularly polymorphonuclear cell) count or local synovial fluid levels of various arachidonic acid products such as prostaglandins or leukotrienes.

(Dr C Dickens)

Sir,

In their study of synovial fluid complement activation Jones *et al*[1] made no assessment of the inflammatory state of aspirated knees. Such assessment could have been attempted using the summated six-point clinical scoring system of Cooke *et al*[2] or by estimation of alternative indicators of inflammation (for example, cell counts, prostaglandins, leukotrienes).

(Dr R Chandler)

Both convey the same message. However, the second is more "punchy" and gets straight to the point by omitting unnecessary description and detail. As with any scientific writing, keep sentences short. Make each of your points separately. Reference short statements rather than provide extended summaries of previous work.

Etiquette and style for letters in response to an article

A letter is the accepted format for comment relating to a previous publication in the same journal. Occasionally it may relate to a publication in another journal.

The usual purpose of such a letter is to offer support or criticism (most commonly criticism) of the rationale, method, analysis, or conclusion of the previous study. If this is the case, make specific, reasoned criticisms or provide additional pertinent data to be considered in the topic under consideration. Do not reiterate arguments already fully covered or referenced in the provoking publication. Your letter should raise points that were not adequately addressed or provide information that supports or refutes the contentions of the other authors. However prestigious you may think yourself, merely offering your personal dissent or approval is not enough. You should use the letter to argue a reasoned perspective. It should not be a vehicle for biased opinion. Always be specific. General comments unsubstantiated by reasoned argument ("I think this a great publication",[66] "I think it's rubbish") are unacceptable.

If offering criticism always be courteous, never rude, arrogant, or condescending. Apart from common decency to fellow investigators, politeness in correspondence will serve to enhance and safeguard whatever reputation you have. This is the same golden rule that applies to question time at oral presentations. No one likes a rude critic, even (or more especially) one who is right. A polite, understated question or comment inevitably has more critical impact than arrogant dismissal. For example, compare the following two styles of presentation. Both letters make the same points.

Sir,

I was greatly surprised that the paper on synovial fluid complement breakdown products (C3dg) by Jones *et al*[1] managed to get into your journal. Firstly, Jones *et al* obviously forgot to control for the inflammatory state of the knees that they aspirated, even though we have previously drawn attention to the importance of this in any synovial fluid study.[2] Secondly, they made no attempt to determine levels of C3dg in synovial fluid from normal knees. Since they only compared findings between rheumatoid and pyrophosphate arthritis knees it is hardly surprising that they jump to the wrong conclusion in stating that complement activation is not a prominent feature of pyrophosphate arthropathy. Thirdly, they only reported C3dg concentrations with no correction for synovial fluid native C3 levels. If these investigators had only taken the time to read the existing literature they would have realised that we previously have shown that such correction is of paramount importance for correct interpretation of C3dg data. That such a majorly flawed paper, which does not even reference our seminal work,[2] should be published at all, let alone as an extended paper, must seriously question the effectiveness of the peer review system that you operate.

A. Pratt

Sir,

I was interested in the study of synovial fluid breakdown products (C3dg) by Jones *et al*[1] in which they conclude, contrary to our previous report,[2] that complement activation is not a feature of chronic pyrophosphate arthropathy. Such discordance most likely relates to differences in clinical characterisation and expression of C3dg levels rather than to estimation of C3dg itself. Unlike Jones *et al*, we assessed and controlled for the inflammatory state of aspirated knees; included normal knees as a control group; and corrected for native C3 concentrations (expressed as a ratio

C3dg/C3), as well as reporting C3dg concentrations. Employing these methods, we were able to demonstrate complement activation in clinically inflamed, but not quiescent, pyrophosphate arthritis knees. Such activation was quantitatively less marked than that observed in active rheumatoid knees. We would suggest that clinical assessment of inflammatory state, inclusion of normal knee controls, and correction for native C3 levels be considered in future synovial fluid studies.

A. Diplomat

Remember that the original authors will usually be invited to respond to your criticisms. It is much easier to respond to a rude than a polite letter and even potentially damning points that you raise may get lost in the "noise" of confrontation. For example, in reply to Dr Pratt's letter Dr Jones would be able to centre his reply around defence of the peer review system. However, he would be hard pressed to sidestep the same specific criticisms levelled by Dr Diplomat. Furthermore, the original authors have the last word and if your criticisms are misplaced (it happens!) you may not be given the opportunity to rescind before publication. You may then find yourself publicly ridiculed, appearing as a rude ignoramus rather than an interested and inquiring intellectual. For example:

Sir,

We are grateful to Dr Pratt for his comments. We had in fact carefully considered all the points he raises. Because all knees included in our study were clinically inflamed, the question of correcting for differing degrees of inflammation does not arise. We also considered aspiration of normal knees but this was not approved by our research ethics committee. We included estimation of native C3 and expression of C3dg/C3 in our original manuscript. This made no difference to the results and because the main thrust of our paper dealt with the method, not the demonstration, of C3 activation in rheumatoid knees (with original data on C4d and factor B activation) we were asked to delete these data by the expert reviewers. We were of course aware of the study by Dr Pratt and colleagues but were limited in the number of references we could include. We therefore referred to the first report of synovial fluid C3dg in normal, rheumatoid and pyrophosphate arthritis knees by Earnest et al[1] which predated that of Pratt et al by six years.

61

Note that letters are always directed to the editor, never to the initial author. The editor in this situation is an impartial intermediary between authors, particularly those in potential conflict.

Box 8.2   Guidelines for a letter in response to an article

- Be courteous and interested, not rude or dismissive
- Make specific rather than general comments
- Give reasoned argument, not biased opinion
- Do not repeat aspects already covered in the original article
- Introduce a different perspective or additional data to the topic
- Attempt to make only one or a very few specific points
- Be concise

Other forms of letter

In many journals the correspondence section is an appropriate site for short reports with a simple message that do not necessitate a full paper. This is particularly true if a study uses standard techniques that are readily referenced and require no detailed explanation.

Presentation of a study as a letter is rather similar to writing an extended abstract (Box 8.3). There should normally be three clear divisions: an introduction relating the rationale and objectives of the study, a section stating the methods and results, and, finally, a conclusion which assesses the validity and importance of the findings in the context of other work. Unlike in concise or extended papers, section headings are not used and an abstract is unnecessary.

Although often considered a "second-rate" way of reporting data, a letter format is quite appropriate for brief reports and can still be prestigious (particularly in certain journals). If presenting original data in a letter, consider carefully whether this will compromise any aspiration subsequently to publish the same data in a more extended form. Remember that letters can be referenced and that "redundant" or dual publication must be avoided.

Case reports are often presented as letters. This is particularly suitable for single cases that do not justify a full or concise report. Some journals have no specific slot for case reports and publish all cases as letters. Most editors only publish cases that give novel

---

Box 8.3 Presentation of a concise report as a letter

- Introduce the topic:
    Briefly explain rationale and objectives of study
- Present methods and results:
    Reference methods as much as possible
    Include only essential data
    Tabulate results if possible
- Present conclusions:
    Emphasise only one or a few major conclusions
    Avoid extrapolating too far from data
- Avoid repetition of data or conclusions
- Be concise

---

insight into pathogenesis, diagnosis, or management. Reporting the sixth case of concurrence of two diseases in the same patient is of no scientific interest – only a formal study, not further case reports, can answer whether this is chance concurrence or a true association that may give clues relating to pathogenesis of either disease. As with short reports, cases are best divided into a brief introduction, description of the case itself, and then discussion of its interest, with no section headings. Be particularly careful not to repeat the same information by summarising the case at the beginning and the end (a common mistake and easy to do).

General or political comment mainly occurs in general journals or specialist journals that are the official outlet of learned societies. In this situation, humorous comments may be permitted. Humour, however, is always risky, especially for an international audience with diverse perspectives on what, if anything, is funny. Letters may be used to advertise an interest in particular cases or investigational material for research purposes or a service on offer (for example, DNA repository). Such advertisements should be very brief and are more usually found in a notes/news section.

9 How to write an abstract for a scientific meeting

R N ALLAN

Introduction

It is, of course, preposterous that anyone should insist that your work, which is at the forefront of scientific development and has consumed your life for the last 12 months, should be reduced to 200 words. Pause, recover your equilibrium, and muster a little sympathy for the organisers of the meeting where you wish to present your original work.

The scientific programme will have been planned several years in advance. The lectures and symposia will have been agreed, the national and international speakers invited, and the venue selected. In addition, the programme will include a limited number of spaces for presentation of abstracts, either as oral communications or posters.

Selection of abstracts

Since the number of abstracts submitted usually exceeds the number that can be included, some sort of selection procedure must be used. A panel of reviewers, expert in their own field, is usually asked to read and mark each abstract. Each reviewer has a large number of abstracts to assess so that the time allocated to read your own precious abstract may well be short. Furthermore, the secretariat organising the meeting will know that authors commonly ignore instructions and submit abstracts over length, illegible, incomplete, and late. They will be determined on this occasion only to consider abstracts which conform to the published guidelines. Be warned!

Guidelines

The instructions may look (and usually are!) tedious but they are designed to ensure high quality reproduction of your work. Abstracts are no longer edited and then typeset. This approach produced well presented abstracts regardless of the quality of the original. For speed and efficiency, abstracts are now photographed and reproduced exactly as they first appeared (camera-ready abstracts). The abstract must therefore be typed within the prescribed area. The appropriate sized typeface and high quality, preferably laser printer should be used to ensure good reproduction. Direct reproduction of the camera-ready abstract will mean that any errors in spelling, grammar, or scientific fact will be reproduced exactly as you have typed them, so take care. Vain hopes that the photographic process might in some way enhance your abstract must be abandoned.

Send the appropriate number of copies. Anonymous copies, without the names of the author and the institution where the work was carried out, are often requested to ensure that the marking system is independent and fair. Make a careful note of the deadline; preparation of abstracts always takes longer than expected. Late entries or those not conforming to the guidelines may be rejected out of hand, without evaluation.

The abstract form commonly includes a number of subject categories and the most appropriate for your work must be noted to ensure that the selected reviewer is an expert in your field. If the choice is available you must decide whether the abstract will be presented as a poster or oral presentation. You will often be invited to declare that the abstract is completely original or submit details if the abstract has been submitted to another meeting or for publication. Full information must be given in a covering letter.

Preparation of the abstract

The abstract should be prepared using a number of headings, even though the headings themselves may eventually be deleted from the final text.

Title

The title is a concise summary of the abstract and must demonstrate that the work is important, relevant, and innovative.

65

Write out the key features of your work and string them together in half a dozen words until the title effectively conveys that message.

Authors

Include authors who have really contributed to the work. It is assumed, if the abstract is accepted, that the first author will present the work. The author presenting the work often has to be identified. The name and address of the institution where the majority of the work was carried out is usually included and the telephone number where the authors can be reached should problems arise. For example, your abstract may be selected for a plenary session when the organisers will need to confirm that the presenter speaks fluent English and that the authors agree that the work is sufficiently important for such a session.

Background

A sentence or two summarising previous work relevant to the presentation is important. Highlight any controversies which your work has helped to resolve.

Aims

What is the point of the study? What is the hypothesis that is being addressed? How is it different from previous work? Is it useful, exciting, and worthwhile? Does it make a new and significant contribution? Encapsulating these ideas in a sentence or two takes practice.

Patients

If patients were studied, how were they selected? Did they give informed consent? Was the selection of patients random? Why were patients excluded? Was ethical committee approval obtained?

66

Methods

The techniques employed must be summarised and novel methods described in greater detail. Minimise the use of abbreviations which only confuses the reader. Note the methods used to test for statistical significance.

Results

Patient data should be described first, including the numbers studied, gender, age, distribution, and duration of follow-up. The key results should then be summarised, usually in four or five sentences identifying the positive features, ensuring that any claims can be substantiated. Highlight new developments.

Discussion

What has the work added to the existing body of knowledge? In what way are these new findings important? Could the findings have occurred by chance or are they statistically significant?

Conclusions

Why is the work important? How might the work be developed further?

From draft to final version

The draft abstract is now complete. It will probably be hopelessly over length. Producing the same information in an abstract of less than 200 words is a real challenge. Delete any duplicated, superfluous or irrelevant information. Can the same idea be conveyed in fewer words? If the abstract is still over length, what are the most important results? Can some be omitted and presented separately at the meeting?

It will take time and many drafts to produce the final version. Start early and plan to complete and submit the abstract well before the deadline. The abstract must summarise the work but do not forget that it must excite the reviewer in that "brief moment of time" when your abstract is assessed.

Re-read the guidelines and ensure that you, your word processor, and secretary have conformed completely with the instructions. Photocopy the original abstract form and ensure that the draft abstract can be laid out effectively within the space available. Circulate the draft abstract to your colleagues and obtain their approval before submission.

Final preparation

The abstract can now be completed and the appropriate number of named and anonymous copies prepared. Do not duplicate submissions – two or more abstracts describing similar results from the same study are both likely to be rejected. You may need to include a self-addressed envelope to learn the outcome of the assessor's evaluation.

Outcome

In due course, you will hear the outcome of the assessment and experience the joy of acceptance or the depression of rejection. Few abstracts are outstanding and few are awful. The marks for most abstracts hover around the mean and are either just accepted or just rejected. Temper the joy of acceptance with modesty. The depression of rejection can be tempered by the knowledge that the abstract was only just rejected.

Presenting the data

The accepted abstract has next to be converted into an oral presentation or a poster – another exciting challenge. Submission of an abstract implies that one of the authors will present the paper or poster in person at the meeting. Late withdrawal of an abstract gives the individual and their unit a bad name.

Conclusion

An abstract which effectively summarises your work clearly and concisely followed by an apparently effortless presentation can only be achieved with meticulous preparation, but in doing so you will sense and share in the excitement of contributing at the forefront of new scientific developments.

10 How to write a case report

J A W WILDSMITH

Case reporting is arguably the oldest and most basic form of communication in medicine. The verbal presentation and explanation of a case history is a skill acquired early in undergraduate training and one that most clinicians use throughout their careers. Much the same ability is required in making a written presentation: the positive features have to be detailed in a sequential and logical fashion, together with that "negative" material that is directly relevant. A case report is, for many clinicians, the first entry into print and, because the basic methodology is familiar, it is a useful exercise in learning to write.

That point made, it is important to remember that all the rules defining other forms of medical writing apply equally to the case report. Clear, unambiguous English should be used to present the material so that the reader has a clear understanding of:

- what happened to the patient
- the time course of these events
- why management followed the lines that it did.

The key feature of a good case report is that it should help the reader to recognise and deal with a similar problem should one ever present itself.

In preparing a case report the writer should be asking three questions:

- What am I going to report?
- How should I report it?
- In which journal shall I aim to publish the report?

What to report

Most doctors occasionally come across a patient whose condition might merit production of a case report. The key is both to observe and to think about clinical practice. In today's circumstances it is a very lucky doctor who describes a totally original condition, but there are many rare or unusual patients who may merit description. However, rarity is not, in itself, cause for publication. The case must be special and have a "message" for the reader. It could be to raise awareness of the condition so that the diagnosis may be made more readily in the future, or the report might indicate how one line of treatment was more suitable and effective than another. What such case reports do, to draw a legal parallel, is establish "case law" for relatively rare disease states.

The second group of patients who may be worth reporting are those with unusual, perhaps even unknown, conjunctions of conditions which may have opposing priorities in their managements. A variation on this theme is the patient who presents with a rare or unusual complication of a disease or therapeutic procedure. Again, though, it is important to indicate what message there is in *this* patient's case for those who read about it. Almost as important as the message is that the case should be interesting to read about. Clearly, skill as an author is going to influence readability, but no amount of writing skill is going to make an uneventful case interesting.

It is as well to remember from the beginning that the first reader of the report will be the editor. Although some editors are totally averse, many feel that case reports help to attract readers by making their journals seem a little more relevant to "ordinary" clinicians who consider that the more scientific contributions do not immediately interest them. Most editors whose journals include case reports receive many more than they have space to publish, so it is up to the writer to ensure that the report is unusual, interesting, and readable so that it is accepted.

Assess the potential response

In deciding whether your case meets the above criteria it is useful to consider how others might respond to the details. A review of the literature may indicate that your case is rare or unusual, but a literature review is time consuming and expensive. It may be more

71

helpful initially to describe the patient to two or three colleagues of varying seniority and see what the responses are. Thereafter, verbal presentation at a departmental meeting will help refine your product. What is rare in one hospital, however, may be commonplace in another because of differences in referral patterns. What seems unusual may be relatively routine elsewhere and sooner or later it will be necessary to do a literature search. It is also necessary to ensure that the motive for publishing the case is not self-aggrandisement. It is the patient who should be interesting, not the author's skill in diagnosis or management.

Many modern case reports describe complications and these can produce a range of responses. Ideally, such a report should make the reader grateful that he or she was not involved, but intrigued at what happened. It should indicate also how the problem can be avoided in the future. However, it is but a small step from here to the reader feeling that somebody (and sometimes everybody) involved in the management of the patient made a complete mess of it. Thus the report may extend a publication list, but do nothing for professional reputation! Conversely, in these audit conscious days we are being encouraged more to "own up" when things go wrong and such reports have merit if the message is clear to others. The *British Medical Journal* encourages this under the general heading of "Lesson of the Week".

How to report

Having established that your case is of interest to others you need to ensure that the material is presented in a fashion that will make others share your interest. It is probably wise to start by writing down (for your initial verbal presentation) the details of the case, then develop the discussion, and finally add the other components. However, this is not the way in which the reader will encounter the report and the overall sequence must be kept in mind throughout.

Title

Most journal readers decide which papers they are going to read by skimming the titles. If the title of a case report is too full the reader may feel that it has said all there is to know. Ideally the title should be short, descriptive, and eye catching.

Authorship

Establishing authorship is an increasing problem in medical publication and this applies particularly to case reports. Only one person should actually write the paper, with the other authors restricted to those who had a significant input to the management of those aspects that were unusual. Thus, a case report written by two or three individuals may be reasonable, but it is difficult to see any justification for a list of five or six authors describing the management of one patient. This smacks of ego "massaging" in the interest of the future advancement of the first named author.

Introduction

There is a tendency to write a short history of the condition when introducing a case report, but this is either unnecessary material or should be put in the discussion. Certainly, the introduction may be used to place the case in context or indicate its relevance, but there is often no need to have an opening section at all. The report may begin simply with the case description.

Case description

In writing the core part of the paper, it is essential to keep to the basic rules of clinical practice. The details will vary a little according to the specialty, but the report should be chronological and detail the presenting history, examination findings, and investigation results before going on to describe the patient's progress. The description should be complete, but the real skill is to accentuate the positive features without obscuring them in a mass of negative and mostly irrelevant findings. Consider what questions of fact a colleague might ask (this is one reason for an initial verbal presentation) and ensure that the answers are clearly within the report. Illustrations can be particularly helpful and in some circumstances they are essential. A photograph of the patient or of the equipment used, line diagrams of operative procedures, graphs of physiological measurements, and summary tables of events can all, when used appropriately, add much to the reader's understanding.

Never forget that it is a patient who is being described, not a case, and that confidentiality must be absolute. Age, occupation, and geographical location might be all that a determined journalist requires to identify the patient, yet such information can be essential to the report. Similarly, blanking over the eyes may be sufficient to obscure identity only if the reader does not know the individual. Increasingly, it may be wise to obtain written consent from the patient at an early stage in the preparation of the report, particularly if photographic material is to be used. Some journals now insist on this.

Discussion

In preparing a report of an unusual condition it is often tempting to expand the paper and produce a review of the literature, particularly if a great deal of work has been put into gathering all the published information on the condition, but it is a temptation that should be resisted (by editors as well as authors). If a review is merited it should be written as an entirely separate exercise by a much more experienced author than is usual for a case report.

The main purpose of the discussion is to explain how and why decisions were made and what lesson is to be learnt from *this* experience. It may require some reference to other cases but, again, the tendency to produce a review must be resisted. The aim should be to refine and define the message for the reader. The good case report will make it quite clear how such a patient would be managed in the future.

References

As indicated, reference to the work of others should be made only where it is necessary to make a clear point. If a standard textbook has indicated that one line of treatment should have been followed, then it should be quoted. Reports by others should be mentioned only where they actively support (or contradict) the particular experience and conclusion.

No matter how exhaustive the search of the literature has been, it is possible that something may have been missed out. It is a very brave, and perhaps foolhardy, author who claims absolute priority in the description of some clinical phenomenon.

Acknowledgments

Acknowledging the assistance and support of others is almost as difficult an area as deciding who should be among the authors of a case report. The key question is whether the patient would have been managed or the paper written without the assistance of that specific individual. A particular problem is deciding whether it is necessary to thank the consultant or other individual clinically responsible for the patient for permission to publish details. With the increasing tendency to seek permission from the patient it would seem that this rather old-fashioned practice can be allowed to die out.

Where to publish

A provisional decision about which journal the report will be submitted to should be made before starting to write. The next stage must be to read the guide to contributors. Journals vary in style and it is helpful to try and picture how the report will appear in print while it is prepared. The author should always aim for a peer reviewed journal and one which he or she already reads regularly. Familiarity with the journal will provide a better idea of what the editor, and thus the readers, find interesting and this will help with the whole process of preparation.

Thereafter, the decision is going to lie between a general, specialist, and even subspecialty journal. The choice will depend on the rarity of the case and its specific features. Keep in mind the basic reason for writing a case report: namely, that it should have a message for the reader. Decide what the message is, consider who the message is aimed at, and then select a journal whose readership will include the target audience.

The final stages of preparation

Once the first draft is written, it should be put away for a week or two, then refined and revised several times. Reading aloud, first in private and later to one or two others who have not heard the case before, is invaluable. This will help improve the clarity of the report and its English as well as bringing out any inconsistencies of fact or interpretation. The text should be checked and rechecked

Box 10.1   Guidelines for a case report

- The report should detail:
    What happened to the patient
    The time course of events
    Why the particular management was chosen
- There may be no need for an opening section. Begin with the case description if possible
- Positive features should be accentuated and irrelevant details avoided
- A photograph or other illustration may be useful
- Confidentiality must be absolute
- The discussion should be useful and not overlong
- Reference other work only when necessary to make a specific point
- Cases that really merit publication always have an educational message

for errors in spelling, punctuation, and adherence to the journal's instructions on style. Finally, the requisite number of clear copies, correctly paginated, should be sent with a polite covering letter to the editor and accompanied by a silent prayer that the next issue of that journal does not contain an identical case!

11 How to write a review

IAN FORGACS

There is no question that the task of writing a review article has become a whole lot tougher over the last few years. The days are surely numbered when it is acceptable for an editor to offer the numero uno top banana in the field a modest (and they always are modest) honorarium in exchange for a few thousand words on the great man's reflections on the contentious areas in his particular specialty. For areas where there is a wealth of valuable data, out has gone the personal perspective and in has come the systematic review as the careful weighing of evidence has surpassed the *ex cathedra* overview – indeed, the very term "overview" carries, for many, a tendency to produce the most astonishing degree of pretension among authors.

There remain, of course, whole areas where there is a lack or, at very least, a paucity of evidence and the more traditional or narrative review retains its place. However, even here, it has become necessary for authors of such reviews to declare the sources on which their opinions are founded.

Who needs review articles?

Journal editors like reviews. The thorough, authoritative review is likely to be widely read and highly cited which may increase the journal's Impact Factor (a measure of a journal's success). Readers also turn to a review article as they feel that, like a morning jog or a cold shower, it might improve them. Market research suggests that, while readers may skim original material, they tend to make the effort to read topical reviews in the unequal struggle to keep up to date. In other words, reading reviews is good for you. Many specialties have journals which consist of little more than a collection

77

of reviews. These are usually worthy but dull. Indeed, many review articles are often quite tedious, although they don't have to be. It is absolutely essential that reviewers transmit the enthusiasm that carries them through the working day. This chapter may help you write an article that might actually be read by someone other than the author, the editor, and the proofreader.

Who should write a review?

Editors will usually try to persuade someone right at the cutting edge of a particular field to provide the article. In general, the further the author is from the frontier of knowledge in that particular area, the less well informed is the review. From time to time, journals receive unsolicited review articles for consideration. In many instances, such pieces read uncannily like the introductory chapter of a thesis or dissertation – and are invariably only too lightly disguised! Editors should spare their readers these unauthoritative and dreary offerings. If you experience the desire to write a review for a particular journal, first go for a brisk walk in a nearby park. If you still feel the need to share your thoughts on a specific topic with the world at large, do make polite enquiry of the editor as to how such a piece might be received before putting pen to paper.

Many journal editors report increasing difficulty in recruiting authors to write reviews. There is no shortage of eminent folk who are only too willing to put together a commentary or leading article of up to 1500 words, but it is becoming harder and harder to persuade the great and the good to write reviews. The likelihood of a reviewer accepting a commission is often inversely proportional to the length of piece required. The mutually acceptable answer may be to accept co-authorship between the desired star name and a less well established colleague. Clearly the junior partner(s) will do most of the real work but an editor can reasonably expect that the finished product represents a real collaborative effort.

Writing a systematic review

Unfortunately, there is some confusion over the meanings of the terms "meta-analysis" and "systematic review" (see Box 11.1). Meta-analysis is, in effect, a piece of research combining evidence from a number of separate studies in a quantitative manner. By

---

Box 11.1

- A meta-analysis is research in which data from separate studies that address a similar research question are quantitatively combined and then statistically analysed.
- A systematic review is a review article based on data from original research studies that have been selected in an objective and rigorous manner using a defined methodology.

---

careful use of original data, meta-analysis has the potential to provide a more precise effect of a particular intervention than can be gained from the results of individual clinical trials.

While meta-analysis can be considered to be original statistical research, the systematic review involves the balanced assessment of original research studies. Conclusions are drawn, not from mathematical summation, but from an objective review of relevant studies which have to meet acceptable criteria of quality. Whereas both meta-analysis and systematic reviewers need to apply rigorous criteria in selecting the appropriate material for their respective endeavours, it is the meta-analyst who goes for a mathematical synthesis, while the reviewer settles for a balanced yet critical summary. The main advantage of being systematic is that the personal views and prejudices of the author are suppressed by the weight of objectivity. In modern jargon, being systematic means being evidence based and such reviews have become increasingly important in a world in which clinical effectiveness is translated into clinical governance.

Finding the data (Box 11.2)

Computerised searches are very helpful but are almost invariably not complete. Access to the large databases such as Medline,

---

Box 11.2　Obtaining the data

- Search through computerised databases – Medline, EMBASE, Cochrane Library
- Personal knowledge of the relevant literature
- Checking the reference lists of papers
- Hand search of the key journals

EMBASE, and the Cochrane Library is readily available in all libraries and in most clinical and academic departments and, increasingly, in the homes of Internet connected medical authors. Searching does take some practice but, with a combination of luck, tact, and charm, your local librarian can be a helpful tutor in search strategy technique. You may really need help to focus on your specific area of interest if your initial search reveals several thousand articles!

Nevertheless, even the best databases are incomplete. Personal knowledge of the field (a *sine qua non* for a reviewer) nearly always throws up articles unrevealed by computer. Checking the references of the various papers is helpful and can be supplemented by a manual search of the title pages of the key journals in the field. Because of publication bias (the tendency for trials with negative results never to see the printed page) a fully systematic search might involve a direct approach to authors to ask if they have (or know of) unpublished data. Such thoroughness would be regarded by most editors as a counsel of perfection, but it would be appropriate to ensure that your review marshalled the data as comprehensively as possible. In particular, it is necessary to emphasise the results of studies which are well designed and this is especially important in assimilating data from clinical trials. It can be very helpful to tabulate the outcome of a series of studies and the merit of such a table is strengthened by giving some indication of those studies that report the results of good quality, randomised, double-blind, controlled clinical trials.

A good review should do more than just present the data and readers expect a reward for their time spent on your prose in the form of some sort of conclusion. Remember that readers who are running out of time or stamina really appreciate a clear summary, most usually offered to them in the form of bullet points.

Writing a narrative review

The systematic review lends itself to specific topics in which there exists a body of data concerning particular intervention(s) in clinical practice – for example, the role of a specific pharmacological intervention in the management of acute myocardial infarction or the value of interventional endoscopy in upper gastrointestinal haemorrhage. Yet there are many areas in which being systematic is just not possible. This may be because there are just no comparative data available or because the whole subject area is not one that can be evaluated by such methodology. One cannot be systematic in a review article on the molecular genetics of breast cancer. However, it is important for the reviewer to amass the key material so as to avoid personal bias in favour of a particular viewpoint. The most serious crime that a review author can commit is to be partial.

Whether being systematic or narrative, the most time consuming aspect of putting together a review article consists of collecting together the source material. If this has not taken up nine tenths of your total expenditure of time on the whole project, then you are either exceptionally well organised, lucky, or insufficiently prepared.

Constructing the article (Box 11.3)

An eye catching title can be a good start but avoid flippancy. A review article on recent progress in extracorporeal shock wave

---

Box 11.3 Constructing the review

- Effective title
- Clear introduction
  what the article is about
  say why it is worth reading
  make it clear you are informed and interesting
- Statement of how the data were selected
- Presentation of data
- Clear conclusions

---

lithotripsy in cholelithiasis can be cheered up by such a title as "Shock news for gallstones". The opening paragraphs are the most crucial in the whole piece. By the end of the first page, you should have explained to the reader exactly what your piece is about, convinced him that the article is worth reading, and demonstrated that what you have to say is informed, authoritative, and interesting. Many otherwise able reviews are condemned to be read by no more folk than can gather together in a phone box because of verbal tedium.

Often the first sentences of any article are the hardest to write and, once a few hundred words have appeared on screen, it all seems rather easier. Although I do not belong to the school of

81

endless drafts and redrafts, there are few final versions of medical articles that have not benefited from radical excision from earliest drafts of the first couple of hundred words – they usually say little and mean even less. My editorial red pen is never wielded more energetically than when the author has failed to follow this guideline.

Medical journals are increasingly formulating quite strict guidelines for authors of reviews. Although there is some danger that, in itself, a standard format can be mind numbingly dull, at least it ensures that the article meets the minimum criteria set by the journal. It is becoming standard practice for the author to be required to state, quite early on in the review, how he selected the information on which the review was based. While journals are, thankfully, still a long way from adopting the view that all reviews must be systematic, they do expect that the author will come clean on how the material was selected. A journal's reputation can be seriously dented by a maverick author basing his piece on a highly selective perspective of the literature.

The body of data should be presented in a form in which justice is done to its level of complexity but notice is also taken of the reader's attention span. A reviewer should think not of his peers in the field but of the averagely intelligent but interested non-specialist (indeed, why should a peer really need to read a review?). The inspired teacher's gift for the helpful pause and reiteration of tricky concepts, aided by judicious use of tables and figures for relevant material, is likely to produce the best review.

It really is a requirement of a good review that the author draws the strands of data together into a conclusion. The reader deserves a few "take-home messages". At all costs, avoid the dreaded final sentence that simply states that all the present studies seem to be in conflict and that more research is needed. You will hear the collective groan of the readership when they get to the end only to find that they are, in reality, rather stuck in the middle. Remember that your review, like most of the really rewarding human endeavours, should end in some sort of climax.

12 The role of the editor

G SMITH

Objectives of the journal

The function of the journal is determined by its editorial board. The editorial board extends to the editor broad guidelines on the type of journal which the editor should produce. For example, the purpose of the *British Journal of Anaesthesia* is the publication of original work in all branches of anaesthesia, including the application of basic sciences. In addition, the journal publishes review articles and reports of new equipment.

The journal may be a weekly or monthly publication of a specialised or general nature. These features may have an important impact on editorial policy – for example, the necessity for specialist assessors' opinions.

Editorial policy

The editor should have formulated a policy for implementing the objectives of the journal.

Policy for authors

The editor should ensure that all correspondence with authors is dealt with rapidly, effectively, and courteously. Assessors' reports should be obtained expeditiously and transmitted rapidly to the authors. in particular, assessors' reports should be detailed, meticulous, and of high quality. if the manuscript is rejected as being unsuitable for publication, the assessors' comments should be seen by the authors to be fair and acceptable.

Policy for readers

The editor attempts to incorporate in each issue of the journal at least some article, be it editorial, original article, book review, or correspondence, that will appeal to any reader of the journal. Articles should be up to date and of high scientific quality, represent the leading edge of scientific progress, and be composed in good English which is as comprehensible as possible to the general reader.[1]

Balance of the journal's contents

Material published in a monthly scientific journal may be classified under the various sections described in Box 12.1. As part of his or her general policy, the editor must determine the balance of contents in each section of each issue of the journal. This is determined to a large extent by the nature of the material submitted to the journal but, nevertheless, the editor does exercise considerable influence on the overall contents of the journal.

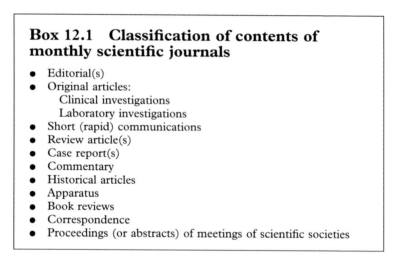

Box 12.1   Classification of contents of monthly scientific journals

- Editorial(s)
- Original articles:
    Clinical investigations
    Laboratory investigations
- Short (rapid) communications
- Review article(s)
- Case report(s)
- Commentary
- Historical articles
- Apparatus
- Book reviews
- Correspondence
- Proceedings (or abstracts) of meetings of scientific societies

Editorials

These may be commissioned as reviews or critiques of original articles accepted for publication in the journal. Alternatively, an editorial may be thought appropriate to describe briefly a subject which does not warrant a full review or to draw attention to very recent innovations. Editorials are particularly appropriate for complementing original articles which either do not present a balanced view of current opinion or require interpretation for the benefit of the general reader.

The editor may publish any number of editorials in each issue of the journal. This distinguishes the way in which different editors imprint their own personality on a scientific journal.

Original articles

These are the mainstay of the monthly scientific journal. The editor may change the character of the journal by policies favouring particular areas of research (for example, changing the balance between clinical and non-clinical research or between basic and applied science) or by encouraging submission of articles in a specific area (for example, intensive care) at the expense of more general articles.

Review articles

These may be either commissioned or uninvited submissions. Again, editors have considerable latitude in pursuing their own policies in respect of the quantity and direction of review material, within the constraints laid down by the editorial board. Editors may decide to subject submitted review material to peer review or take their own decisions on the quality of such articles.

Case reports

These often present considerable difficulties to the editor. In a monthly scientific journal with a low acceptance rate for submitted articles, particularly stringent criteria may apply. For acceptance in the *British Journal of Anaesthesia*, case reports must present a unique problem or reiterate a problem of outstanding importance – for example, relating to anaesthetic mortality.

Other categories

In addition to the above categories, other material may be accepted under a variety of headings – apparatus, laboratory investigations, equipment, history, commentary, etc. Again, the decision to accept such material and the balance of articles reflect editorial policy.

Book reviews

There is little doubt that book reviews are informative and often sought out more avidly by readers than other sections of the journal. Invariably, such reviews are obtained only by invitation; unsolicited reviews are always rejected.

Correspondence

The correspondence section of the journal is extremely important and the editor will attempt to encourage lively and informative debate. Usually, most correspondence relates to published articles in the journal. This section may also be used for floating new hypotheses and particularly for drawing attention to important hazards, because the submission to publication interval is shorter for this section than any other in the journal. The correspondence section should not be used for abbreviated case reports or shortened original investigations which attempt to avoid peer review.

Organisation of the editorial team

Manuscripts submitted to a monthly peer reviewed scientific journal are normally processed by a team rather than a single individual. The editor (occasionally termed the editor in chief) determines the way in which his or her team functions.

Essentially there are two major methods of organising the editorial team (Fig 12.1).

In system (A) the editor acts as the sole final conduit between acceptance of manuscripts in the editorial office and onward transmission to the technical editor or publishers.

In system (B) several individuals may act as conduits between submission of manuscripts and transmission to the publishers. In this system, manuscripts relating to particular subspecialties may be handled semi-independently by section editors – for example, in anaesthesia there may be section editors for manuscripts covering the specialties of intensive care, obstetric anaesthesia, pain, cardiac anaesthesia, etc.

These two types of editorial organisation have specific advantages and disadvantages. In the first system, there is greater uniformity of criteria for accepting and rejecting manuscripts and greater uniformity in subediting; the disadvantage is a much higher

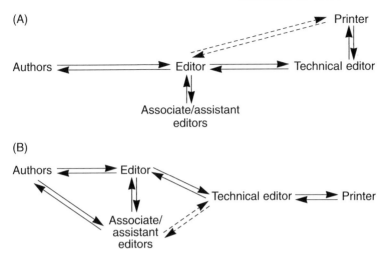

Figure 12.1   Organisation of the editorial team. In the first mode (A) the editor is the sole conduit of communication with authors and technical editors. In the second mode (B) associate editors (or section editors) may be given full responsibility for processing manuscripts.

workload for the individual editor. In the second system, the workload is spread between several individuals and such editors may exhibit greater insight within their own specialised fields; however, the disadvantage is greater lack of uniformity of acceptance criteria and editing.

Processing of manuscripts

Initial screening

Before seeking expert assessors' views on the manuscript, the editor should ensure that some basic formalities have been completed.

● The manuscript should conform to the uniform requirements for manuscripts submitted to biomedical journals.[2] In this agreement, it is stated that a manuscript must be accompanied by a covering letter signed by all authors of the manuscript. The letter should include information on prior or duplicate publication, or submission elsewhere, of any part of the work.

87

- There should be a statement of financial or other relationships that might lead to conflict of interests.
- There should be a statement that the manuscript has been read and approved by all authors.
- The name, address, and telephone number of the corresponding author should be noted.
- Each manuscript should be presented in the standard format (Box 12.2).

Box 12.2   Typical layout of a scientific manuscript

- Title page
- Summary, including key words
- Introduction
- Methods
- Results
- Discussion
- Acknowledgments
- List of references
- Tables (including legends to tables)
- Legends to illustrations

Pages should be numbered in the top right hand corner, the title page being 1, etc.

The editor also initially ensures that the contents of the manuscript are appropriate for his or her particular journal. For example, if the journal is a predominantly clinical one, manuscripts relating to basic laboratory investigations may automatically be returned to the authors without formal assessment.

Assessors' reports

After the initial screening, the editor seeks expert advice on the quality of the paper. Advice may be sought from one, two, three, or occasionally more expert assessors. The assessor is asked particularly if the work is original and if the experimental methodology is sufficiently accurate and reproducible to generate data on which sound conclusions may be based. Advice may be offered to the assessors in the form of standard guidelines (Box 12.3). Assessors may be asked to produce an anonymous report for transmission to the author and also to complete advisory guidelines confidential to the editor.

Review of assessors' reports

Armed with the benefit of assessors' advice and his or her own review of the manuscript, the editor may draw one of three conclusions.

- The manuscript is unacceptable for publication and is unlikely to be modified in such a way as to become acceptable for publication. Often the major reasons for this decision are that the work is not original or that the methods of investigation are inappropriate or inaccurate. It may also become clear at this stage that the material is not appropriate for the particular journal.
- The manuscript is acceptable for publication either as it stands or with some minor modifications.
- The present manuscript is not acceptable for publication but that it *might* become acceptable subject to modifications. To guide the authors as to the extent of modifications required, the editor may send them the assessors' confidential reports together with a covering letter (which may incorporate comments made by the assessors on the confidential report). In addition, guidance may be provided on the statistical handling of the data and editorial changes which may be required to produce conformity with the style of the journal.

The revised manuscript

The editor may decide on his or her own initiative that the manuscript is acceptable for publication or (with the benefit of clarification of questions of originality or methodology) that the paper is quite clearly unacceptable for publication. If additional expert advice is required the editor may seek further reports from the original or new assessors.

Editorial decision

It is important to emphasise that the assessors' reports represent only guidelines for the editor and they do not dictate the editor's

Box 12.3 Guidelines for reviewers*

1 The unpublished manuscript is a privileged document. Please protect it from any form of exploitation. Reviewers are expected not to cite a manuscript or refer to the work it describes before it has been published and to refrain from using the information it contains for the advancement of their own research.

2 A reviewer should consciously adopt a positive, impartial attitude towards the manuscript under review. Your position should be that of the author's ally, with the aim of promoting effective and accurate scientific communication.

3 If you believe that you cannot judge a given article impartially, please return the manuscript immediately to the editor with that explanation.

4 Reviews should be completed expeditiously, within 2–3 weeks. If you know that you cannot finish the review within the time specified, please inform the editor to determine what action should be taken.

5 A reviewer should not discuss a paper with its author.

6 Please do not make any specific statement about the acceptability of a paper in your comments for transmission to the author, but advise the editor on the sheet provided.

7 In your review, please consider the following aspects of the manuscript as far as they are applicable:
   Importance of the question or subject studied
   Originality of the work
   Appropriateness of approach or experimental design
   Adequacy of experimental techniques (including statistics where appropriate)
   Soundness of conclusions and interpretation
   Relevance of discussion
   Clarity of writing and soundness of organisation of the paper

8 In comments intended for the author's eyes, criticism should be presented dispassionately and abrasive remarks avoided.

9 Suggested revisions should be couched as such and not expressed as conditions of acceptance. On the sheet provided, please distinguish between revisions considered essential and those judged merely desirable.

10 Your criticisms, arguments, and suggestions concerning the paper will be most useful to the editor if they are carefully documented.

11 You are not requested to correct deficiencies of style or mistakes in grammar, but any help you can offer to the editor in this regard will be appreciated.

12 A reviewer's recommendations are gratefully received by the editor, but since editorial decisions are usually based on evaluations derived from several sources, a reviewer should not expect the editor to honour his or her every recommendation.

* These guidelines were prepared by the Council of Biology Editors.

course of action. Editorial decisions are based upon editorial policy, assessors' reports, the assessors' confidential comments to the editor, the editor's reading of the manuscript, the flow of manuscripts to the journal, and constraints imposed by the size of the journal. As only a relatively small proportion of manuscripts may be instantaneously deemed acceptable or unacceptable for publication, the editor may rely heavily upon his or her judgment of what represents an advance on our current state of knowledge and the degree to which confirmation is required. For example, when a new drug is introduced for the treatment of a particular disease it is important that several centres, probably in different countries, provide confirmatory evidence of the pharmacological and therapeutic action of that drug. However, there comes a time when additional studies are not required and then they may be rejected on the grounds that they do not represent an advance in our current state of knowledge.

Editing the manuscript

After accepting a manuscript for publication, the editor may either edit the manuscript himself or herself or pass it to an associate editor for this purpose. The process of editing follows certain principles.

- An attempt is made to shorten the manuscript without any loss of accuracy. Authors often repeat data in the results and discussion section of a manuscript. Repetition is common in a concluding paragraph or, indeed, if a summary is appended to the manuscript. In my experience, the most common form of repetition is where the same data appear in both tables and figures (often because the figures have been used as part of a verbal presentation to a learned society).
- Where manuscripts have emanated from non-English speaking countries, considerable effort may be required to correct English grammar.
- The editor may change phrases or sentences to standardise to a particular "house style" – for example, use of the term "tracheal tube" rather than "endotracheal tube".
- The references may be checked for accuracy and validity.

91

- The manuscript is standardised in respect of drug names, symbols, units, and abbreviations. Frequently, this work is undertaken by a professional subeditor (or technical editor).

Technical editing

Having finished with the manuscript, the editor passes it with a disk to a technical editor who edits the disk on screen and introduces notations required to produce the correct fonts and lay out of the manuscript when it is produced by a computer controlled printing press.

Proof stage

Proofs from the printer are sent to the technical editor, the authors, and the editors, all of whom make corrections. These are passed on to the technical editor, who collates the corrections and transmits a corrected disk to the printer.

Page proofs

Final page proofs are seen usually only by the editor and technical editor.

Publication

It will be clear from the foregoing that the process of publishing a scientific manuscript is complex and time consuming (Fig 12.2). For a monthly journal, therefore, it should be anticipated that many months will elapse between submission of a manuscript and its eventual publication.

Other published material

As the editor is responsible for assessing every word that appears in the journal, it is necessary for him or her to review all material, including advertisements, for both commercial and academic purposes. Commercial advertisements must be closely vetted to ensure that outrageous claims or inaccuracies are avoided and academic advertisements assessed for accuracy insofar as it is possible.

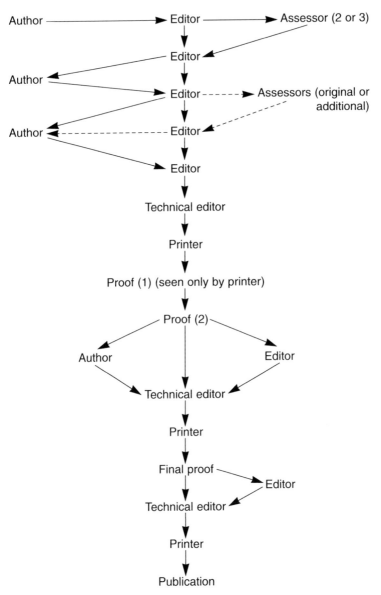

Figure 12.2   Stages in the progress of a manuscript from submission to publication.

Postscript

The rejection rates of leading monthly journals such as the *British Journal of Anaesthesia* may exceed 60%. Editors may therefore have to deal with aggrieved potential authors and unsympathetic reviewers exhibiting the same range of emotions as proud parents whose offspring have been abused by their teachers. An important role of the editor therefore is to act as an impartial referee imbued with tact, sensitivity, and insight. The lot of an editor who does not strive to attain these qualities is not a happy one!

1 Extended guide to contributors. *Br J Anaesth* 1990;**64**:129–36.
2 International Committee of Medical Journal Editors. Uniform requirements for manuscripts submitted to biomedical journals. *BMJ* 1988;**296**:401–5.

13 The role of the manuscript assessor

STEPHEN G SPIRO

I spent five years as an editor of a scientific journal during which I did no reviewing for other journals but carefully evaluated hundreds of reviewers' assessments and recommendations as to whether a manuscript should be accepted or not. I was always pleased to see comprehensive, positive, and helpful reviews which would not only make my job easier but would also be of great value to the prospective authors, whether the manuscript was accepted or not. Even a rejection with constructive, valid reasons for this decision can be of considerable help to authors when rewriting their paper for submission elsewhere.

The most important factor in assessing a manuscript is time – something few of us have in abundance. In retrospect, I did my best work for the journal when on holiday, sitting on a balcony high in the Swiss Alps among a ring of large, snowy mountains with an immense feeling of wellbeing after a good day's hiking. Here, time stood still and reviewing was easy and almost a pleasure. I am back on the same balcony three years later musing what the perfect manuscript reviewer should do.

Of course, in the normal way of things, the only time a reviewer feels pleased or even flattered to be asked to assess an original manuscript is the first time.

The role then becomes an unpredictable one, with more papers thrust upon one the more established or expert in a field one becomes. Usually, individual editors keep a computer database on how many manuscripts an individual reviewer has at any one time, and try not to overburden. The system can break down, however, if the associate editors of a journal board select reviewers independently and select the same individual without their colleagues' knowledge. Furthermore, the well known "professors of original ideas" will get requests to review from a range of journals within a specialty and this is hard to take into account.

Reviewers, therefore, should not become overloaded and editors should establish the number of manuscripts an individual may wish to assess in a year. At the same time, the reviewer should, on receiving a manuscript, decide whether he or she has the time to assess the paper. If not, return it immediately. Nothing is worse for an editor, or, of course, the authors, than a potential reviewer who sits on a manuscript for several weeks and then decides that he or she is too busy. It is also not acceptable to just pass the manuscript to a junior colleague and then send their assessment back with a brief covering letter as if the requested reviewer has really performed the critique.

Secretaries should be primed to push a request for a review under the boss's nose and not into the "to do" pile as a precious week could elapse before the manuscript is even noticed. Holidays and lecture trips are another problem – the secretary should at least inform the enquiring editor that Dr A is away for two weeks and ask whether the manuscript should be returned or not.

A useful system that some journals employ is to fax the potential reviewer with the top sheet and abstract of a manuscript and ask for a return fax as to whether the reviewer is prepared to do the work within the stipulated time. If so, the whole manuscript is sent.

Who should be a reviewer?

That's easy! The best and most authoritative in that field. The problem is that Professor Best and Famous is likely to be far too busy, usually abroad, and too involved in writing his or her own papers and grants to enjoy lots of reviewing. Furthermore, there could be conflict in that the paper sent for review represents the efforts of the competitors within the field. Can one be totally unbiased, not lift their ideas, and provide timely, positive, and fair assessments?

In practice, much of the above is not a problem, apart from finding time to spare. Most authorities are very honest and dispassionate and provide constructive reviews. The difficulty is to establish how much time they are prepared to commit. A good editor will soon learn to comply with the reviewer's capacity.

If the head of a department is not available – where next? Research fellows, especially those who have already published in the field, can be superb. They are full of the latest knowledge on a subject and, once they have learnt to be neither defensive nor aggressive about another potential contribution to "their" field, they can provide the best reviews. In essence, the important thing is to look widely for reviewers, including abroad. Most established scientists and physicians world wide will provide excellent reviews in English and a journal will soon build up its database of good, reliable individuals.

Box 13.1   A conscientious reviewer should:

- Confirm without delay whether he or she can or cannot review the article within the stipulated time
- Make arrangements to inform an editor if the manuscript arrives when he or she is away
- Inform the editor for whom he or she reviews most frequently how many articles a year he or she can deal with
- Have the ability to be objective and unbiased in his or her comments
- Not pass a manuscript to junior colleagues without informing the editor

---

The review

Perhaps the worst, most unhelpful review is the one that is late, comes after desperate faxes and 'phone calls, and states, "This is a well written manuscript with an important message, clearly argued, and should be accepted".

This usually means that the manuscript has been glanced at, not critically assessed, and, in my experience, the original manuscript that fulfils these comments has yet to land on my desk. The two line review makes it almost impossible for the manuscript to be rejected (if this is the recommended decision) without a huge amount of work either by the other reviewer (if one is fortunate) or by the editor. The editor or associate editor has to maintain the reviewing standard of the journal and often has to produce an additional review if a reviewer lets him or her down.

Most journals pass across to the other reviewer the assessment received from the second reviewer along with the final verdict and the reasons that took the editor to this decision, so that the reviewer can assess his or her comments in light of those of a colleague. We are all vain enough to hope that our review was the one that contained the real reasons for rejection/acceptance but, if not, there is the chance to learn from other colleagues and the editor's assessment. If the two line reviewer does not buck up, he or she will not be used again.

On receiving a new manuscript, it is almost impossible to avoid noting from whom and where it came. This, many feel, biases the reviewer. One is less likely to reject a manuscript from Professor Best and Famous than the first manuscript in the field from a little known author or a new group of researchers. There has been considerable controversy as to whether reviewers should be aware of the source of the manuscript, but this debate remains to be settled. Once you start the manuscript, read it through from beginning to end. Assess the style; does it correspond to that of the journal? If not, the paper may have been prepared for another journal and already rejected. Your version may not have been altered – a tell-tale sign of sloppiness – or the authors have not bothered to discover the style rules for your journal. These are irritating irregularities, perhaps more likely to be picked up by an editor than a reviewer, but, if the authors cannot be bothered to put the manuscript into the style of a particular journal, it makes the reviewer less likely to try very hard.

Is the manuscript *title* of interest and does it reflect the content and thrust of the paper? Clearly, if the manuscript is not making a point or not presenting data of sufficient interest or importance, it is unlikely to succeed. Occasionally, the manuscript is better than its title and the reviewer should consider rewording the title more appropriately.

How many *authors' names* are on the manuscript? Again, the editor may become concerned if the number is large and may wish to be reassured that each has made an important contribution. However, the reviewer is likely to be more expert in the area of a particular manuscript than the editor and comments as to the acceptability of six or more potential authors are of inestimable value for the editor.

The *language and style* of a manuscript greatly influence its digestibility and clarity of message. The reviewer must make allowances for those who are not writing in their native tongue. Whilst non-English speaking authors are advised to get an English speaking colleague to read a manuscript before it is submitted, many do not and the results are very mixed. Minor linguistic blemishes can be dealt with but if the English is so opaque that it is open to misinterpretation, then the manuscript should be returned with the request to rewrite it, emphasising the particularly unclear sections. It could then be resubmitted.

During the initial read through, it is helpful to note errors, typos, and minor queries on a separate sheet or PC (do not mark the manuscript itself). These points can be added later as a list to the overall assessment. These often minor comments are both helpful to the editor and the author, and also reassure the author that you have actually thoroughly read the paper.

The *abstract* is the most important part of the manuscript. It should state clearly why the study was done, what the results were, and what conclusions were reached. Ambiguity or confusion here, or a dubious reason for performing the study, will probably set the reviewer against the document.

The *introduction* should allow the reviewer to understand why the study was performed, what the gap in knowledge was, and why. There should be a succinct argument for the paper and some, not too much, justification, by referring to other related work in the field. Is there *really* the gap in knowledge that the authors claim, that is, is this a worthwhile project, irrelevant, or perhaps a reinvention of the wheel?

The *methods section* is very important and most reviewers make their decisions here. One must hope that the reviewer is up to date in the subject, especially if methodology is complex or novel. However, the presentation, validation, and extrapolation of the methods chosen have to be presented in such a way that they are clear, likely to be correct, and can be repeated elsewhere. Serious doubt should render the paper unacceptable. The reviewer also needs to be satisfied that the number of subjects or tests performed are of sufficient magnitude or accuracy to give the result adequate statistical power. The literature is full of articles containing results on small numbers of patients or other data, with inadequate statistical power for firm conclusions. These papers will suggest something is likely or possible, but not probable or definite. The reviewer must decide if the paper contains sufficient data to make the conclusions probable.

The question of how subjects were selected for the study needs careful thought. The reviewer must be satisfied that there was no selection bias or suspicion of undisclosed reasons for not selecting certain subjects and that randomisation (if present) was correct. There should also be a statement that an ethical committee has approved the study.

Finally, the methods section must summarise the statistical tests chosen. Many reviewers are not as familiar with statistics as they would wish. If in doubt, the reviewer should consult a statistician colleague and clearly state in the report that this has been done and include the usually very helpful comments of the statistician. If a statistician has not been involved and the reviewer has some reservations, the editor must be informed in the covering letter when the review is returned.

The *results section* should clearly summarise the relevant data. Many authors do this badly with much repetition in the text and often further repetition in the tables and figures. The reviewer should ensure that the presentation of the results is clear, logical, and contains all correct p values. Many indigestible data can best be summarised in tables or figures. The reviewer can greatly improve the clarity of the manuscript here. Check that tables are not too large and overwhelming. Also, check that they are not too small, when perhaps a sentence in the text will sometimes suffice, or whether two small tables can be combined.

All figures and tables should stand on their own, that is, have clear titles with legends for abbreviations used and significant differences readily visible and comprehensible.

The *discussion section* is unlikely to influence the decision to accept the paper. Nevertheless, it is an important one and should clearly summarise the results, contain a critique of the methods used, comparisons with other work in the field, have a clear conclusion, and, perhaps, pose questions for further work. Most discussions are too long, too defensive, and often repeat much that was contained in the introduction. A good reviewer can decide what is relevant and what can be deleted. Also, points missed by the authors, such as relevant papers not mentioned, should be requested. Usually, a discussion can be shortened considerably.

Finally, the reviewer should look through the *references* to ensure that the important papers in the field are listed and to check spellings of names. The editor can advise on style if necessary.

Having worked through the manuscript section by section, the question of style may remain. If a paper is scientifically good enough, but poorly written, it is greatly appreciated if the reviewer would attend to the major problems. The editor and ultimately the technical editor will correct simple linguistics. However, major changes of language or suggested reordering of sentences or even paragraphs could be made to everybody's benefit by the reviewer at this stage. The editor will not have sufficient time to correct the style of all papers likely to be accepted. However, if a manuscript is returned to the authors with a conditional acceptance, the authors should deal with language and presentation problems. If the reviewer makes suggestions and corrections, not only does this help the editor but it means a much improved revised version will return and require less work before, hopefully, final acceptance. The revised manuscript is unlikely to be seen by the reviewer.

Whilst the final decision is the editor's, the reviewer should give a clear indication in his covering letter to the editor as to whether a paper is acceptable for publication or not. Most scientific journals accept 30–40% of original manuscripts and most of those are only accepted subject to adequate revision. If a paper seems likely to be accepted, the reviewer must carefully list the areas that need revision, those that need correcting or improving, and those that need expanding or shortening. The reviewer will probably have a list of queries, suggestions for improving the manuscript, and occasionally a request for further additional work to ensure that the claims in the manuscript are substantiated. These comments should be provided in a logical sequence together with all minor corrections. If a manuscript is rejected and the authors receive comments from a reviewer including the advice that the manuscript should be accepted, this will often lead to difficult correspondence; hence, keep the review relatively dispassionate. Editors have several reasons for rejecting a manuscript which include not only scientific grounds, but also pressure of space, originality, similarity to another recently published or accepted article, etc.

The peer review system seems to work extremely well as the great majority of reviewers are generous with their time, provide detailed and constructive comments to keep both the editor and authors happy, and supply the type of detailed effort that they would expect to receive themselves on a paper of their own submitted for publication.

Ultimately, being asked to review for a respected scientific journal is, in itself, a form of recognition of the reviewer's standing in the field and is something that they most readily respond to. Many reviewers acknowledge this by citing journals that they have reviewed for in their CV. It seems to be a self-perpetuating system that works in general to a very high standard indeed.

Box 13.2   Important points to remember

- The title and number of authors are appropriate.
- Is the manuscript submitted in the style of the journal?
- Does the abstract succinctly explain the aims, methods, and results, and have a clear conclusion?
- The introduction should explain why the study was done, with some appropriate references to relevant literature.
- The methods section should be clear, contain validatory data, and be reproducible elsewhere. The methods of enrolling subjects should be free from any potential bias. The statistics should be comprehensible and the study sufficiently large for statistical power.
- Results should avoid repetition in text, tables, and figures.
- The discussion should summarise the main findings, criticise methods used, relate to other data in the literature, and form effective conclusions.
- The discussion can usually be shortened.
- Reviewers should separate major criticisms and suggestions for revision from minor errors, changes, and other textual amendments.
- The report should not include a recommendation for acceptance or rejection.
- Correction of language and rearrangement of text as necessary are of great help to the editorial team.

---

14 What a publisher does

ALEX WILLIAMSON

Congratulations! Your paper has been accepted for publication.

At this point, the author may have his or her first contact with the publisher. In most cases this will be a fruitful collaboration, but many authors have only a vague notion of what a publisher actually does. This is evident because of the number of times I am asked, "What exactly is it that you do?".

Authors write and the publishers provide the means for those authors to reach their audiences. The services a journal publishing house offer fall into a number of broad categories, some of which an author will have no direct contact with but nevertheless cannot do without. The categories are: editorial, production, fulfilment, distribution, sales and marketing, and finance. Each category is dependent on the others and all work closely together.

Editorial

Within the editorial department there are two main functions – managing and commissioning and copy editing.

Managing and commissioning editors

Managing and commissioning editors (also called publishing managers, acquisitions editors, or sponsoring editors) are the publishers' representatives to journal editors, learned societies, and authors. The main function of a managing editor is the care of the existing list of journals. This consists of financial management, liaison with the learned society (if one is involved), overseeing the duties of the copy editor, production, advertisement sales, marketing, subscription fulfilment and distribution, and, last but by no means least, liaison and support of the journal editors. These editors are a rare breed of dedicated professionals who are often full time clinicians or academics or both. For little or no reward, they devote many hours to editorial work and need strong support from the publisher.

Managing editors will also receive new journal proposals, seek specialist opinion via both questionnaires and personal contacts, analyse, research the market, cost the proposal, and, finally, present it to their management. The rejection rate for new journal proposals is very high indeed – roughly speaking, only one in ten proposals will be successful. A new journal launch requires a large investment from the publisher and so a decision to launch is never taken lightly.

The managing editor will meet the editor regularly and offer advice on publishing practice and will help in the training of support staff for the editorial office. The editor should be given a realistic budget to cover the costs of running the office in terms of postage, telephone and fax, stationery, photocopying, and secretarial assistance. Most editorial offices now run a computerised manuscript tracking system which streamlines much of the peer review procedure.

Once a manuscript is accepted for publication, the editor will send it as hard copy or on floppy disk to the publisher where it will receive the attention of the copy editor.

Copy editors

Copy editors (also called technical editors, subeditors, or production editors) provide the main link between an author and the publisher. The copy editor will prepare the accepted manuscript for press. These days increasing use is made of the author's word-processed file. Usually at the acceptance stage, the author is requested to provide his or her manuscript as hard copy and as a word-processed file on floppy disk. The majority of copy editors are now fully computer literate and will do all the necessary editing of the author's file on screen. Some copy editors still prefer to edit on the hard copy but the publisher will usually require that these amendments are recorded on the floppy disk as well. These electronic files will then be automatically translated into the appropriate format for the journal. The days when manuscripts were completely rekeyed at the typesetters are probably gone for ever. These changes have meant that the copy editors have learned new skills and in many cases will be adding tagging and codes to the word processed author file which will enable the page make up programme to operate seamlessly and take in the artwork, figures, and tables, which will also have been generated electronically. In addition to the word processed and tagged file used to generate pages, the files will also be stored electronically for reuse on the Internet, on CDs, etc. The copy editor will also be scrutinising the tables and illustrations.

Copy editors will adapt the manuscript to the "house style" of the journal. They are concerned with details of style and ensure that spelling, grammar, punctuation, capitalisation, and mathematical conventions follow approved practice. They also look for accuracy and consistency. They pick up loose ends, discrepancies, omissions, and contradictions. Substantive queries may be referred back to the author and editor at this stage. More often, the problems identified are minor and will appear as queries to the author on the proof. Copy editors will suggest relettering and redrawing of illustrations where necessary and will size them and place them appropriately in the text.

Copy editors will liaise with the supplier and ensure that proofs are distributed quickly to authors and editors. They will read the proofs and collate any corrections received from authors and editors. Only in exceptional circumstances are authors allowed to make major changes to their papers at this stage and the copy editor will refer substantive author corrections for the editor's approval.

Copy editors work to tight schedules and will often need to remind authors to return proofs promptly.

In collaboration with the editor and the advertisement department, copy editors make up the contents of each issue and pass final proofs for press. At this stage the publishing process passes to the production department.

Copyright

Either at acceptance of the manuscript for publication or at the proof stage, the author will be required to assign copyright to the journal. Publishers are much better able to defend copyright than individual authors and will act on their behalf.

With the advent of electronic publication, many publishers will ask the author to assign the rights for electronic and print editions.

Offprints

Offprints are extra copies of the articles which are printed at the same time as the journal issue. At proof stage authors will also be given the opportunity to purchase a quantity of offprints of their paper. This used to be a very popular service for authors but the ease of photocopying has almost eliminated the need for it. Many publishers now provide a free copy of the relevant journal issue to the corresponding author instead of providing free offprints.

Production

Very few journals now use conventional typesetters but instead will send their edited electronic files to an originating house (usually part of a major printing house) where the edited text files are married with the artwork, tables, and figures and the pages are generated and proofed. The production staff will choose appropriate printers for the journal, bearing in mind the budget, print run, schedule, and the use of colour illustrations and advertisements. They choose and purchase text paper and cover boards. The production department is responsible for schedules, obtains estimates, and controls costs. It keeps abreast of the latest advances in print and bind technology and will advise editorial colleagues on appropriate new means of production which will benefit the journal in terms of schedule, cost, and appearance. Overall, the production team is responsible for the look of the journal, its cost-effective production on schedule, and delivery for onward distribution to the subscriber.

Fulfilment and distribution

The average specialist journal's circulation is subscription based, usually on an annual basis. By and large, subscribers fall into four main categories.

1   Institutional or library subscriptions at the full price subscription rate. Most of these sales are handled via subscription agents, who make the librarians' jobs much

simpler. Librarians will probably deal with only one agent for the thousands of subscriptions they purchase. The agent will consolidate these orders and deal with the individual publishers, quite often using computers to facilitate the transfer of orders. For this service agents are given a discount by the publishers.

2 Personal subscriptions at a discounted subscription rate.

3 Member subscriptions. Often a journal will be owned by or published in association with a learned society. The annual membership subscription will include an automatic subscription to the society's journal.

4 Free and exchange subscriptions. The editor and editorial board will normally receive free copies. Copyright legislation decrees that journal issues must be deposited in the British Library and several other major libraries. Subscriptions are given to the large abstracting and indexing services such as *Index Medicus*, *Current Contents*, and *Excerpta Medica*.

All these groups expect to receive the journal regularly and on time and subscribers need to be reminded each year to renew their subscriptions. Most subscription fulfilment systems are computer based and will generate mailing labels sorted into postal categories to a defined schedule. In many cases, these mailing labels will be despatched directly to the printer, who will arrange onward posting to subscribers. In other cases, publishers will handle all distribution from their own warehouses. Overseas consignments are often sent in bulk by air to a mailing house, which then organises onward distribution by that country's mail service. The warehouse will store additional copies of the journal to fulfil claims for missing issues, back orders, and single copy sales.

With the advent of electronic publishing, some of the major journals are offering full text versions for online access or are producing CD-ROMs which are available at the completion of the volume. At the time of writing, there are a multiplicity of access options available ranging from free online access for all through free access for current subscribers to the hard copy version to access on payment of an additional amount to the subscription to the hard copy. We live in changing times and who knows what will happen eventually. However, most publishers are confident that journals have a future; we just do not know in what form that will be!

Sales and marketing

The main source of revenue for a journal comes from the sale of paid subscriptions. However, there are other sources and I shall deal with these first before returning to the subscription area.

Advertising sales

The higher circulation general and specialist clinical journals enjoy a good revenue from the sale of display advertising space in each issue. The major space buyers are the pharmaceutical companies but equipment manufacturers and publishers also use journals to advertise their products.

The advertisement sales team not only maintains close links with agencies and companies but also liaises with the editorial team. A strong editorial policy on the percentage of advertisement versus editorial pages is needed together with a strict code on the permitted content of advertisements and their location in comparison with editorial pages. Despite these safeguards, editors and publishers are often criticised about the content and placement of advertisements. Nevertheless, advertisements can provide a useful service to the reader and certainly support the journal financially.

Reprint sales

Reprint sales can be a considerable source of revenue, particularly where papers are reporting the results of clinical trials or new indications for an existing drug. Reprints should not be confused with offprints. Offprints are printed simultaneously with the journal and are primarily given free or sold at cost to authors. Reprints are produced later, usually in bulk, and are of necessity more expensive and appeal to the commercial sector.

Rights

The marketing of a journal involves not only the sale of subscriptions but also the sale of subsidiary rights. These may take the form of translation rights, rights to produce an English language edition in a slightly modified form for a foreign market, or rights to produce cheap reprints in countries where purchasing power is low.

Bulk and single copy sales

Occasionally a journal will publish a special issue or supplement on a particular "hot" topic and this may attract bulk sales from a commercial organisation or single copy sales to individuals.

Subscription sales and marketing

When a new journal is launched, the circulation climbs steadily and then plateaus as the journal becomes established in its specialty. Some people are of the opinion that once a journal has reached its plateau it is no longer necessary to continue active promotion. Not so! Every year an established journal will lose some 10% of its circulation owing to consolidation of library collections, budgetary restrictions, or simply a change in the direction of research in the institution. To maintain its circulation, a journal needs to be promoted to pick up new subscribers to replace those that have been lost.

In collaboration with the subscription and fulfilment department, the lapsed subscribers will be actively encouraged to renew their subscriptions and ultimately will receive a questionnaire which can provide valuable information to editorial colleagues.

The marketing department is concerned with promotion material, publicity, and advertising. It devises campaigns to promote each journal and designs, writes, and produces leaflets and catalogues which are sent by direct mail to specialists and librarians world wide. Apart from direct mail, journals are promoted via advertisements in other relevant high circulation journals and displays at appropriate specialty meetings and symposia.

The Internet is now used as a very effective marketing tool which can reach a large target audience very cheaply and, if managed well, can provide useful details of the types who visit the site often. Most of the major publishers have websites and many journals have their own individual sites. Usually details are given of the editor and editorial board, current and archived contents, instructions for authors, and where and how to subscribe.

Finance

The staff of the finance department have a number of roles – all of them concerned with money! They raise invoices, control cash flow, maintain records, and pay suppliers. The management accountant will provide monthly accounts to the senior management and will play an integral part in the constitution of annual budgets and longer term strategic planning.

Conclusion

The role of the publisher has been compared with a variety of functions, few of them favourable. We have been told we are parasites, middlemen, gamblers, to name but a few. Perhaps we are best regarded as catalysts who facilitate the communication between the authors and their readers.

15 Who should be an author?

RICHARD HORTON

Regrettably this question is impossible to answer. Five years ago, I could have confidently referred you to the standard definition provided by the International Committee of Medical Journal Editors (otherwise known as the Vancouver Group) (Box 15.1).[1] All was clear back then. The criteria that had to be satisfied for you to qualify as an author (to be, shall we say, Vancouver Group positive) were unambiguous.

And they needed to be. Authorship is the currency of academic life. Citation provides the intellectual credit that fuels promotion and career success; it gives an independent estimate of a researcher's contribution to science. Authorship is the foundation of our system for judging academic value and assigning reward.

Before I ruin this picture of serene harmony, I should point out that most biomedical journals adhere to the Vancouver Group definition.[2] Their editors will require you to be Vancouver Group positive. In other words, to confirm in either a covering letter or a separate signed statement that you fulfil the Vancouver definition. You are likely to say you do even if you know that you or a co-author do not. To provide your signature confirming that you qualify as an author is something you do automatically, perhaps without even thinking very much about the implications of what you are doing.

Nowadays, though, the certainty that editors of leading medical journals once possessed lies in shreds. Our happy consensus has been destroyed. Following a conference on authorship in biomedical science, held in Nottingham, UK, in 1996,[3] first *The Lancet*[4] and then the *British Medical Journal*[5] abandoned the Vancouver Group definition (although their editors are part of the Group). In its place we put the concept of contributorship,

111

Box 15.1   How to be a Vancouver Group positive author

All persons designated as authors should qualify for authorship. Each author should have participated sufficiently in the work to take public responsibility for the content.

Authorship credit should be based only on substantial contributions to: (1) conception and design or analysis and interpretation of data; (2) drafting the article or revising it critically for important intellectual content; and (3) final approval of the version to be published. Conditions 1, 2, and 3 must all be met. Participation solely in the acquisition of funding or the collection of data does not justify authorship. General supervision of the research group is not sufficient for authorship. Any part of an article critical to its main conclusions must be the responsibility of at least one author.

Editors may ask authors to describe what each contributed; this information may be published.

Increasingly, multicentre trials are attributed to a corporate author. All members of the group who are named as authors, either in the authorship position below the title or in a footnote, should fully meet the above criteria for authorship. Group members who do not meet these criteria should be listed, with their permission, in the acknowledgments or in an appendix.

The order of authorship should be a joint decision of the co-authors. Because the order is assigned in different ways, its meaning cannot be inferred accurately unless it is stated by the authors. Authors may wish to explain the order of authorship in a footnote. In deciding on the order, authors should be aware that many journals limit the number of authors listed in the table of contents and that the US National Library of Medicine (NLM) lists in Medline only the first 24 plus the last author when there are more than 25 authors.

an idea first described by Fotion and Conrad[6] but developed more fully by Drummond Rennie and colleagues.[7 8] This shift away from traditional notions of authorship is the most important recent crack to appear in the architecture of academia. It has the potential to threaten the entire structure of modern science. Why? And where does that leave you, someone who simply wants to get your work published?

First, most scientists ignore editors and most so called authors are likely to test Vancouver Group negative. For example, Shapiro et al[9] found that a quarter of the "authors" they surveyed contributed nothing or to only one aspect of the published work. Eastwood et al[10] discovered that a third of the US postdoctoral fellows they questioned were happy to list someone as an author even if he or she did not deserve it, provided that the inclusion of their name would make publication more likely. Given this widespread cynicism about the meaning of authorship, to cling to a definition that no one uses seems crazy.

There is a second, more sensitive reason for questioning our existing beliefs about authorship. Several recent instances of scientific fraud[11][12] have revealed that the flipside of authorship *credit* – namely, authorship *responsibility* – is often overlooked. When individual researchers have their names listed on the byline of a paper, it can be difficult to dissect out who did what if an aspect of the work is questioned. Instances of fabrication or falsification of data have revealed the importance of assigning the precise and explicit parts played by individual investigators in a research project.

These two forces make it hard to resist two ensuing interpretations. First, that researchers should be allowed to list whoever they wish on the byline of a paper, Vancouver Group positive or negative. And second, that editors should ask for and publish a clear description of the contributions made by the authors. Rigid, unenforceable, and widely ignored definitions should be abandoned. This is the new policy of the *BMJ*[5] and *The Lancet*.[4] The *BMJ* has gone further than *The Lancet* and asks each group of contributors to select one or more guarantors who will take overall responsibility for the integrity of the entire work.

The reaction to contributorship has been mixed. At *The Lancet*, we have found that most authors readily accept the idea that contributors should be cited at the end of each paper (Box 15.2). But some have voiced concerns that unethical authorship practices – inappropriate credit in the form of guest authors or the unacknowledged contributions of ghost authors – are likely to continue.[13]

Still, other journals are likely to follow the move to contributorship. Even if contributors lists are not always embraced, the principle of complete disclosure and personal responsibility is accepted.[14] You need to be aware which journals prefer traditional Vancouver Group positive authors and which prefer contributors. For all practical purposes, you can freely ignore the rules set by the former group. Everybody else does.

An additional issue that also defies easy rules is the acknowledgment section of your paper. Whom you choose to thank

---

Box 15.2   An example of contributorship

Byline: A, B, C, D, E, F, G, H

Contributors: A carried out the trial, helped in data analysis, and wrote the paper. B was involved in design, implementation, and data analysis, and contributed to the writing of the paper. C was involved in execution of the trial, data management and analysis, and quality assurance of the turnip assay. D was involved in trial execution and data entry, management analysis, and quality assurance. E was involved in trial execution and data management with emphasis on analysis. F and G were involved in the design and contributed to the writing of the paper. H was involved in the design, implementation, analysis, and biochemical interpretation, and contributed to the writing of the paper.

[Guarantors: A and H]

Box 15.3   Acknowledgments according to Vancouver

At an appropriate place in the article (the title page footnote or an appendix to the text; see the journal's requirements), one or more statements should specify: (1) contributions that need acknowledging but do not justify authorship, such as general support by a departmental chair; (2) acknowledgments of technical help; (3) acknowledgments of financial and material support, which should specify the nature of the support; and (4) relationships that may pose a conflict of interest.

Persons who have contributed intellectually to the paper but whose contributions do not justify authorship may be named and their function or contribution described – for example, "scientific adviser", "critical review of study proposal", "data collection", or "participation in clinical trial". Such persons must have given their permission to be named. Authors are responsible for obtaining written permission from persons acknowledged by name, because readers may infer their endorsement of the data and conclusions.

Technical help should be acknowledged in a paragraph separate from that acknowledging other contributions.

can be impossible to separate from whom you choose to cite as an author on the byline. Not surprisingly, the Vancouver Group has something to say about acknowledgments (Box 15.3). The likelihood is that contributors lists and acknowledgments will eventually fuse and the whole subject of academic reward based on research contributions will be overhauled.[15]

Given this confusing state, there is only one rule to bear in mind when deciding who is an author, a contributor, a guarantor, or an acknowledgee. Decide who is to be what *before* you start your study. Most authorship disputes arise when the work is completed and a paper has to be written. Then comes the jostling for a place (and position) on the byline. Primary prevention is always better in the end.

1 International Committee of Medical Journal Editors. Uniform requirements for manuscripts submitted to biomedical journals. *Ann Intern Med* 1997;**126**:36–47.
2 Parmley WW. Authorship: taking the high road. *J Am Coll Cardiol* 1997;**29**: 702.
3 Horton R, Smith R. Signing up for authorship. *Lancet* 1996;**347**:780.
4 Horton R. The signature of responsibility. *Lancet* 1997;**350**:5–6.
5 Smith R. Authorship is dying: long live contributorship. *BMJ* 1997;**315**:686.
6 Fotion N, Conrad CC. Authorship and other credits. *Ann Intern Med* 1984; **100**:592–4.
7 Rennie D, Flanagin A. Authorship! Authorship! Guests, ghosts, grafters, and the two-sided coin. *JAMA* 1994;**278**:469–71.
8 Rennie D, Yank V, Emanuel L. When authorship fails: a proposal to make contributors accountable. *JAMA* 1997;**278**:579–85.
9 Shapiro SW, Wenger NS, Shapiro MF. The contributions of authors to multiauthored biomedical research papers. *JAMA* 1994;**271**:438–42.
10 Eastwood S, Derish P, Leash E, Ordway S. Ethical issues in biomedical research: perceptions and practices of postdoctoral research fellows responding to a survey. *Sci Eng Ethics* 1996;**2**:89–114.
11 Lock S. Lessons from the Pearce affair: handling scientific fraud. *BMJ* 1995; **310**:1547–8.
12 Marshall E. Fraud strikes top genome lab. *Science* 1996;**274**:908–10.
13 Greenfield B, Kaufman JL, Hueston WJ, Mainous AG, De Bakey L, DeBakey S. Authors vs contributors: accuracy, accountability, and responsibility. *JAMA* 1998;**279**:356–7.
14 Editorial. Games people play with authors' names. *Nature* 1997;**387**:831.
15 Horton R. The unmasked carnival of science. *Lancet* 1998;**351**:688–9.

16 Style – what is it and does it matter?

NORMA PEARCE

What is style?

"Style" has a number of meanings, at least two of which are relevant to the writing and publishing of scientific papers.

First, it refers to a manner of expression in language. "Have something to say and say it as clearly as you can. That is the essence of style," urged Matthew Arnold, while Jonathan Swift firmly believed that "proper words in proper places make the true definition of style".

Style may also be defined in more specific terms as the custom followed in spelling, capitalisation, punctuation, and printing arrangement and display – the house style.

The foreword to my copy of the *JAMA Stylebook* states that "a scientific journal should have a consistency of style and an accuracy of reporting on which readers come to rely. The few rules a journal adopts should be simple, inviolable, and encourage clear unambiguous writing". There follow approximately 160 printed pages of simple, inviolable rules – which might lend credence to the view (albeit somewhat extreme) that house style is the accretion of the personal prejudices of generation upon generation of nit-picking obsessionalists! Yet the *Economist* stylebook became a bestseller so consistency, clarity, and accuracy (nit-picking?) must be widely recognised as desirable qualities in a piece of writing.

Style creates a favourable impression

These days, it seems, researchers are under great pressure to publish their work – careers and funding depend on publications as never before. Articles pour into journal offices. A few are of

---

Box 16.1   Does style matter?

- Style matters for its own sake; standards are important
- Style is necessary for the efficient dissemination of medical knowledge
- House style gives individual publications their identity
- Attention to style can count when it comes to having papers accepted

---

great scientific value, some are poor, and most are middling fair. Articles in the first two categories are generally easy to spot, but editors spend a great deal of time deciding which of the "middling" articles merit publication. Undoubtedly, good writing style and attention to detail can improve the chances of an "average" article being selected for publication.

Instructions to authors

Editors are human enough to be favourably impressed by a clear, easy to read paper whose authors have paid heed to the journal's "Instructions to contributors". Very few authors seem to read these. Journals do have different styles, which can be tedious for an author who has to rework an article each time it is submitted to a different journal. But it is sensible, and good manners, to set out a paper as requested and use the correct style for references and units (errors occur when results have to be converted and references changed from Harvard to Vancouver style or vice versa). All this effort also makes life less traumatic for authors, since even the most pedantic subeditor warms to the well presented paper and becomes more sparing in his or her use of the subeditorial pen.

Some elements of style

Good style, like good English, is not easy to define and it is much easier to say what it is *not* than what it *is*. I will not discuss spelling, punctuation, or capitalisation here because these aspects of house style do not usually result in open warfare between the author and subeditor. More "creative" subediting may cause problems, however, so I have listed below some "do's and dont's" that should help reduce these.

117

Keep it short

- Editors are biased in favour of short articles (and short reference lists) as space is at a premium.
- If it is possible to cut out a word or sentence, always do so. "Now" is better than "at this moment in time" and "agreed" is better than "came to the identical conclusion".
- Sometimes whole paragraphs are redundant: the introduction often tells readers what they already know and results should not be repeated in the discussion section.
- A law exists (somewhere) which states that the piece of prose of which you are most proud is probably the bit that should go first!

The longer the sentence, the greater the likelihood of confusion

Long sentences can make laborious reading. "The relatively short duration of action on serum gastrin of SMS 201-995 when compared with omeprazole was also observed in our study since on the day after the five day treatment serum gastrin levels were increased due to the prolonged effects of omeprazole on gastrin release" is easier to follow if it is written as two sentences. "Our study also showed that the effect of SMS 201-995 on serum gastrin was not as long lasting as that of omeprazole. Serum gastrin concentrations were still high the day after a five day course of omeprazole treatment."

Syntax may go adrift in complicated sentences, tenses can become confused, and verbs and subjects may not agree when they have become lost or long separated in an overambitious construction.

Never use a long word when a short one will do

Writing scientific articles is not the same as writing "link lines" for Edwardian music hall. Long, complicated words will irritate rather than impress readers and do not make for easy reading.

Polysyllabic words do not have greater scientific credibility – "bifurcation" is not a more grown up word than "fork".

Avoid figures of speech and idiom

Scientific journals have an international readership. Write in a way that can be understood by someone whose first language is not English.

Passive constructions should be used sparingly

Passive constructions can be very dull. Use the active voice. "I love you" has much more impact and immediacy than "You are loved by me" and it's two words shorter!

Avoid foreign, technical, or jargon words

If you can think of an ordinary English word use it. "The patient could walk" is better than "the patient was ambulatory"; "arms and legs" is preferable to "upper and lower extremities".

Words and phrases often used in medical conversation, such as "full work up" (investigation) and "blood sugar" (blood glucose concentration), are best avoided in writing.

Use abbreviations with care

- Abbreviations that are current in one country may not be recognised in another.
- Take a paper with lots of abbreviations, spell them all out in full, and some rather odd constructions may become evident.
- Well known abbreviations such as ECG, AIDS, and CT are permissible, but papers littered with unfamiliar, distracting abbreviations can be difficult to read.
- Always spell out an abbreviation the first time it is used.

Prepositions are better than strings of nouns

- Do not let a desire to cut words obscure the meaning of what you write.
- Lists of nouns (noun salads) as in the title "Doctor workload reduction programme" might cause difficulty to someone whose first language is not English; "Programme to reduce the workload of doctors" is longer but easier to understand.

Watch prefixes

The prefix "un" seems to be disappearing in favour of "non". Perhaps some people think that "non" has a more scientific air, but in many instances its use is incorrect. Thus we have "non-treated" patients, subjects given "non-necessary" drugs, and even "non-transplant immunological diseases".

Danglers

Make sure that modifying words and phrases refer clearly to the word modified. In the sentence, "Seven hundred and sixty patients were treated at St Mary's Hospital between 1964 and 1991 with azathioprine", poor old azathioprine is dangling around rather helplessly.

Participles do not provide a strong opening for sentences and hanging participles, as the next sentence illustrates, lead to ambiguity: "Having a high temperature, one of us gave the patient a tepid bath" (the high temperature applies to "the patient" and not to "one of us").

Structure can improve effectiveness

Go through your piece of writing underlining the subjects of clauses and sentences and then the most important sentence in every paragraph. Sentences that begin with the subject are easy to understand. Putting the key sentence at the start of the paragraph is more effective than leaving it to the end or hiding it in the middle. If underlining shows that your pattern is consistently different from this, try to restructure your sentences and paragraphs.

Edit your own paper first

The job of the subeditor is to make the paper conform to the house style of the journal and to prepare the script for the printer. Contrary to the view of some authors, subeditors do not really like to rewrite, but sometimes this is necessary because of poor English or lack of clarity. Although it can be very annoying to have sections of a paper rewritten by a subeditor, especially if this seems to change the meaning, it is possible that the message was not absolutely clear in the first place.

Most of us have great difficulty in being objective about something we have written – because we know exactly what we mean, we imagine everyone else will. It may be worth trying to appraise an article from the viewpoint of a subeditor before it is submitted for publication.

- Distance yourself from your writing – do not look at it for a few days, then reconsider it stringently. Time can be a problem for those (most of us) who set deadlines then leave things until the last minute and do not have the few spare days required for this exercise.
- Record yourself reading the article aloud, then play back the recording. This should help to pinpoint any clumsy constructions.
- Ask a trusted friend or colleague to go through the paper querying points she or he does not fully understand; any ambiguity can then be rectified before the paper is subedited. (Let us hope the same can be said for the friendship.)

By this time you may be so bored with your article that you do not care what happens. Be resolute, be bold, post it ... and remember Charles Lamb's words, "When my sonnet was rejected, I exclaimed, 'Damn the age; I will write for Antiquity' ". That's style.

17 Ethics of publication

MICHAEL J G FARTHING

Introduction

This is a new chapter for *How to Write a Paper* but it is far from a new topic. Ethical considerations have taken centre stage in the protection of the rights of patients and healthy volunteers in research studies and in considering the welfare of animals used in biomedical research. Medical ethics has found a clearly defined position in most undergraduate medical curricula. Ethical issues relating to research integrity and the publication of research findings have lagged behind, despite the apparent increase in the number of detected cases of serious research misconduct in North America, Europe, and elsewhere.

I came face to face with publication ethics when I became editor of *Gut*, a specialist journal for gastroenterology and hepatology.[1] In my first year we detected redundant publication (an attempt to publish data the majority of which had been published in another journal in the preceding year), "salami slicing" (publishing a study piecemeal when a single, high quality paper would have been preferable), outright plagiarism, and papers submitted without the knowledge or consent of co-authors. Compared to the major cases of fraud that have come to light in the last year or so, these are minor offences and all were detected before publication. Retractions were therefore not required and no author faced public disgrace. However, they raised important questions for me as the editor and, I hope, for the individuals concerned when their actions were discovered. Unlike some countries in the world, the United Kingdom has no regulatory agency that deals with research misconduct although the most serious cases are reported to the General Medical Council (GMC), usually resulting in a judgment of serious professional misconduct and removal from the GMC register.

There is a feeling among editors and some investigators that research misconduct has become more frequent during the past two decades. It is difficult to be certain whether this perceived increase is a true increase in the number of misdemeanours *committed*, but there is no doubt that the number of serious cases of research misconduct that have been *detected* has increased during this period. Stephen Lock, a past editor of the *British Medical Journal*, has documented known or suspected cases of research misconduct in the UK, the USA, Australia, Canada, and other countries.[2] In the UK, many of the cases involve fabrication of clinical trial data, most commonly by general practitioners although hospital clinicians have been guilty of similar offences. Fraud in laboratory experimentation appears less common, although there have been a number of notorious cases in the USA and UK when the results of laboratory experiments have been fabricated, falsified, or misrepresented.

Research misconduct in the modern era is often considered to have started with William Summerlin, an immunologist at the Sloan–Kettering Institute in New York, who in 1974 used a black felt-tip pen to colour patches of transplanted skin in white mice! Others have claimed to have isolated cell lines from human diseases but subsequent work showed that they came from a monkey. In another example, radioactive iodine rather than phosphorus was used as the "read out" in gel electrophoresis in an attempt to show an important new mechanism in carcinogenesis. The examples are endless. Reports of major plagiarism continue to be detected, as does misrepresentation of personal credentials in curriculum vitae.

What is publication ethics?

Publication ethics is an "umbrella" term covering the many processes involved in research and the publication of results (Table 17.1). Relevant areas range from the most serious aspects of research fraud to the criteria required for authorship and conflict of interest in research publications. Editors must also be concerned by ethical issues associated with the reviewing process and the legitimacy of product advertising in their journals. For the author, publication ethics can be considered under two major categories: research integrity and publication integrity.

Research integrity must be uppermost in the investigator's mind during the conception, design, and execution of a research study.

Table 17.1   The A–Z of publication ethics

- Advertising
- Authorship
- Confidentiality
- Conflict of interest
- Editorial freedom
- Editorial integrity
- Media
- Patient privacy
- Peer review
- Redundant publication
- Research ethics
- Research integrity
- Supplements
- "Whistleblowers"
- Zeal – excessive

It is a multistep process and ethical considerations occur throughout. At the initiation of the research process there should be a protocol which has been reviewed and approved by contributors and collaborators. Research integrity spans study design, collection and collation of results, data analysis, and presentation. Failure amounts to research misconduct which can be regarded as a continuum ranging from errors of judgment (that is, mistakes made in good faith) to what have been regarded as minor misdemeanours, so called "trimming and cooking", through to blatant fraud, usually categorised as fabrication, falsification, and plagiarism (Table 17.2).

Table 17.2   Research misconduct

Errors of judgment	Inadequate study design
	Bias
	Self delusion
	Inappropriate statistical analysis
Misdemeanours ("trimming and cooking")	Data manipulation
	Data exclusion
	Suppression of inconvenient facts
Fraud	Fabrication
	Falsification
	Plagiarism

Publication integrity begins with the writing of the paper. Common examples of failure to meet acceptable standards usually centre on inappropriate or "gift" authorship, redundant (or duplicate) publication, when all or a substantial part of the work has been published previously, and plagiarism, in which text is "lifted" directly from another publication. Full declaration of any conflicts of interest is vital to encourage authors to ensure balance in their discussion and conclusions and to facilitate peer review. Conflicts include direct or indirect financial support from the study, consultancy agreement with a study sponsor, the holding of any patents relating to the study, and any other mechanisms by which financial benefit might accrue as a result of publication of the study. The tendency to attempt to identify "the minimal publishable unit", sometimes referred to as "salami slicing", should be discouraged.

Editors have other ethical concerns, particularly about the quality of peer review and conflicts of interest that might arise in the review process. Additional concerns relate to sponsored supplements to the journal and the influence that advertising by the biomedical industry and others might have on journal content.

Who commits research and publication misconduct?

Research misconduct has been committed by the most junior research fellow and the most eminent research boss. However, the culprits appear to fall into two broad groups. First, there is the relatively naïve, inexperienced investigator, often a general practitioner, who fabricates clinical data usually by adding fictitious patients to a randomised controlled trial. In some instances the motivation is financial, driven by the knowledge that the more patients recruited to the study, the greater the reward. Suspicions are commonly alerted when a particular centre or investigator is able to recruit many more patients than other centres in a multicentre study, has data that are unusual and inconsistent with other centres, and has an increased number of adverse drug events. Detection usually occurs during the monitoring process when clinical report forms cannot be matched to patients' clinical records.

The second category of fraudster is the bright, often young laboratory scientist who succumbs to the pressure for academic success and promotion and the institutional demands to secure research funding. Such individuals are usually medically qualified, male, and working in a distinguished institution with a successful and productive research group. The individual almost invariably has a curriculum vitae that is growing at a rate well beyond that normally expected from an individual at that stage in his or her research career. Research data may be fabricated completely or "massaged" or supplemented in a way that may be extremely difficult to detect. Individuals working in the same laboratory often suspect misconduct but are generally disinclined to come forward as the "whistleblower".

How can we prevent research and publication misconduct?

The widespread nature of research and publication misconduct in all its forms and degrees of severity indicates that existing control measures are inadequate. Improved methods for the detection of misconduct are required, as is the increased vigilance of research supervisors, laboratory co-workers, and editors and all those involved in the publication process. Even if "policing" of research were made more effective, it would not address the fundamental issues as to why some individuals advertently or inadvertently betray their responsibilities as a scientist or clinical investigator. Clear guidance on ethics should be emphasised during research training and in all institutions that are actively involved in research. This should be accompanied, however, by endorsement of the research ethos of quality rather than quantity. A variety of other interventions may also assist (Table 17.3).

The key step in the prevention of research and publication misconduct is education. Institutional guidelines should be available to all researchers as they join a new institution and formal instruction in research and publication ethics should be part of research training and a component of all taught and non-taught courses.

The research

All laboratory and clinical research should be protocol driven. The protocol should be agreed by all contributors and collaborators in the project and their roles clearly defined before the work is begun. It is extremely helpful if authorship is defined at this stage to avoid any conflicts after the study has been completed. The International Committee of Medical Editors (the Vancouver Group) has produced guidelines on authorship which demand that each author must have contributed substantially throughout the

Table 17.3 Can research and publication misconduct be prevented?

Education	Research training
	Research ethics
	Publication ethics
The research	
Protocol driven	
Establish contributors and collaborators	Define roles
	Agree protocol
	Agree presentation of results
Define methodology for data analysis	Statistical advice
Ethical approval	
Project and personal licence (Home Office)	
Supervision	Guarantor
	Communication
	Ensure good clinical practice
	Record keeping
The publication	
Disclose conflict of interest	
Disclose previous publications	
Approval by *all* contributors	
Submit to one journal at a time	
Assume research data audit	

Table 17.4 Authorship (from reference[3])

Authorship credit should be based only on substantial contributions to:

- conception and design or analysis and interpretation of data; *and*
- drafting the article or revising it critically for important intellectual content; *and on*
- final approval of the version to be published.

The three conditions must all be met. Participation solely in the acquisition of funding or the collection of data does not justify authorship. General supervision of the research group is also not sufficient for authorship

process[3] (Table 17.4). "Gift" (honorary) authorship is to be deplored. It is advisable to define and agree the methodology for data analysis before the research begins, to avoid the criticism that bias has been introduced in the way in which the results are presented by selecting an analytical approach that feeds the prejudices of the authors. Statistical advice should be taken during the design phase of the study, not at completion when it is impossible to influence study design. It is unethical to perform a study in which the design is inadequate to answer the question posed.

Studies involving patients or human volunteers must have the approval of the local research ethics committee. Experiments involving animals must be approved by the Home Office and must be covered by a project licence. Individual investigators must in addition hold a Home Office personal licence.

Close supervision of a research project is an essential component of research integrity. Research misconduct may be more prevalent when investigators are isolated, possibly believing that "they can get away with it because no one else will know". Inadequate review of raw data by the project supervisor may facilitate falsification or fabrication in large prestigious departments when a young investigator feels excessive pressure to produce. It has been proposed that there should be a move away from "authorship" towards contributorship and a guarantor who would take overall responsibility for the project.[4] Whatever system is felt to be right, research integrity is dependent on good communication between contributors with frequent discussion on the progress of the project and openness about any difficulties encountered in adhering to the research protocol. Protocol changes should be agreed by all. "Good clinical practice" guidelines should be adhered to in all clinical studies. Record keeping must be of the highest quality. By law, case report forms from all clinical trials and other clinical studies must be kept for 15 years. Laboratory investigators must keep records of all experiments performed which include original data printouts and any other paper or photographic record of experimental results. These should be attached to the appropriate page in a laboratory notebook. Laboratory research records should be retained in the department in which the work has been performed and be available for review for at least 15 years.

The publication

The contributor or contributors responsible for providing the first draft of the manuscript should have been identified at the inception of the study. All authors must have the opportunity to revise the manuscript and all should approve the final version submitted to a journal. If any part of the study has been reported previously, this should be disclosed to the editor of the journal. Any conflicts of interest should also be disclosed when the manuscript is submitted. This should include a clear indication as to how the study was funded and whether any of the authors have any consultancy agreements or patents pending that could influence the presentation and interpretation of the data. Authors should also state whether there are any other direct or indirect ways in which they might benefit financially from the study.

All material presented in the paper should be original. Although "imitation may be the greatest form of flattery", taking text from other published works without acknowledging its source is plagiarism and amounts to research misconduct. Audit has become an essential component of clinical practice and may well be adopted by the scientific community to assure quality of published work. I believe that all contributors to scientific papers should assume that they may be asked to present raw data to validate a research paper. It is possible that journals may randomly audit a percentage of all papers accepted for publication.

What is the editor's role?

Editors are the custodians of scientific literature. They have responsibility for maintaining high standards in research and publication ethics. They depend heavily on the advice obtained through the peer review network which itself may need overhauling. A system which allows the reviewer to know the author of the paper but conceals the reviewer's identity from the author may not be the most reliable or ethical approach to obtaining this advice and there has been a call for complete openness in the peer review process.[5] Reviewers may also have conflicts of interest regarding the paper they have been asked to review, which of course must be disclosed.

Editors have a responsibility to minimise redundancy in the published literature, a task which has been greatly assisted by the coming of the electronic age. Many reviewers, for example, now routinely check research databases to determine whether a paper or a related paper has been published previously. Some editors now argue that this should be the first step before a new manuscript is allowed to enter the journal's editorial process.

Editors do, however, face a major difficulty when they discover research or publication misconduct. Until recently, most editors would merely reject the paper, pointing out, when the evidence is clear cut, that there is plagiarism or redundancy. The editor has no power to carry out an indepth inquiry or sanction any form of punishment. Some editors, however, have indicated to authors that they would not be willing to consider another manuscript for a finite period of, say, 3–5 years, although when publication has occurred then retraction of redundant or plagiarised material is necessary and the authors are then subjected to the inevitable public disgrace. There is a growing feeling among editors that their duty should go beyond this and that the discovery of research or publication misconduct, even if it is prevented, should be reported back to the offender's institution.

What should you do if you suspect misconduct?

Informal surveys suggest that many investigators have suspected colleagues of research misconduct. There is reticence to make such accusations against a colleague because of the inevitable personal difficulties that might result, irrespective of whether the accusations were eventually found to be true. There is innate dislike in the biomedical scientific community of being a "whistleblower". However, information derived through this route is an important way of detecting scientific dishonesty and thus, at least in the early stages of an investigation, the informant should be protected by anonymity. This of course has disadvantages in that it might encourage a malcontent colleague to make accusations behind the screen of anonymity, which ultimately may be shown to be false. The Royal College of Physicians has indicated that every institution should have its own system to manage complaints of scientific misconduct and has suggested a procedure for taking the process forward.[6] The USA, Norway, Denmark, and other European countries have established national agencies to deal with research integrity. Currently, in the UK, the General Medical Council has the responsibility for considering cases of research misconduct among clinical investigators.

1 Farthing MJG. Research misconduct. *Gut* 1997;**41**:1–2.
2 Lock S. Research misconduct: a résumé of recent events. In: Lock S, Wells F, eds. *Fraud and misconduct in medical research*, 2nd edn. London: BMJ Publishing Group, 1996:14–39.
3 International Committee of Medical Journal Editors. Uniform requirements for manuscripts submitted to biomedical journals. *Ann Intern Med* 1997;**126**:36–47.

4 Smith R. Authorship: time for a paradigm shift? *BMJ* 1997;**314**:992.
5 Smith R. Peer review: reform or revolution? Time to open up the black box of peer review. *BMJ* 1997;**315**:759–60.
6 Working Party. *Fraud and misconduct in medical research. Causes, investigation and prevention*. London: Royal College of Physicians, 1991.

18 The future: electronic publishing

MAURICE LONG

The first edition of *How To Write a Paper* was published in 1994. The concluding chapter was entitled "The future: electronic publishing". It contained just one reference to the Internet, the only one in the whole book, and none at all to the World Wide Web. The four years between the first and second editions have seen a sea change in the way science publishing – and almost every other form of communication – is conducted. When the Hubble space telescope is multiplying our knowledge of the cosmos at a greater rate than at any time in the history of science, and when unimaginable progress is being made in the world of genetics, it might seem one hyperbole too many to say that the emergence of the Internet and its World Wide Web in the mid-1990s is the most significant change in the way we communicate since Gutenberg invented movable type in 1455. Some say it is even more significant.

In human endeavour, either in social change or in technical innovations, revolutions occur when a number of related or even apparently unrelated phenomena fuse into something larger than the sum total of all the components. In the previous edition of this book I analysed the "future" by looking at economic, technical, and cultural imperatives. In one sense, the future is happening now, insofar as we are seeing the Internet unfolding before our eyes and it might be instructive to analyse its relevance to scientific communication in the same way

The economics of the Internet

The popularity of the Internet is very largely explained by its apparent cheapness. The billions of dollars spent by the US Defense Department on its earlier incarnation have long since been written off. For the first 20 years of its existence, the Internet proper was managed within the not-for-profit, tax dollar-funded university system in the USA, and this has shielded all its users from its true development and maintenance costs, adding to the perception that it is an intrinsically cheap medium. Local telephone calls in the USA, the home of the Internet, are frequently free and so, for many American users, the Internet seems almost as free as the air that we breathe.

The technology of the Internet

Perhaps the only brand new, brainwave invention in the history of man was the wheel and axle; all else is somehow derivative. The discovery of silicon technology paralleled developments in digital technology and from them both emerged computers – first the bulky mainframes and later the bijou but hugely more powerful personal computers. Neither could work, of course, without operation and application software, the "languages" that enable machines to talk to us and to each other. The digital bits and bytes stored in the computer are nothing more than electrical impulses until they are assembled and interpreted and perhaps even spoken by the software, like the thousands of random pitches and frequencies rescued from chaos by the genius of Mozart to form the wondrous Clarinet Concerto.

Charles Babbage built his Difference Analytical Engine in London in the 1820s; in 1844, Samuel Morse sent his first commercial telegraph. It took a further 150 years for data management and communication technologies to merge to form the Internet's World Wide Web. When they met, they lifted each other to an altogether higher value than either could ever have achieved separately.

The culture of the Internet

The Internet has changed the technology and even the conventions of communication for ever. It started in 1887 when Emile Berliner produced the first disc recordings of classical vocalists. The ability to listen to the Clarinet Concerto at home was unimaginable before Thomas Edison invented the phonograph for dictating speech. Then, as in a whirlwind, came moving pictures, mass radio, television, video recorders, compact disks. The Internet, or more accurately its World Wide Web, is the inevitable and logical extension of all the miracles worked by Edison, Marconi, Logie Baird, Sam Goldwyn, the scientists at CERN, and Bill Gates. Apparently cheap, easy, and fun to use.

The Internet might be changing the promulgation and publication of science research more profoundly than anything since the first appearance of the *Philosophical Transactions of the Royal Society* in 1663. For most people involved in the science communication "chain", however, it is very difficult to understand fully what is happening now and where it will lead to. Those managing the communication flow, especially publishers and librarians, must at least attempt an analysis and try to plan for the near future. Those with imagination and luck might be able to forecast the medium term future as well (five to seven years); only prophets and visionaries can see beyond. And yet, some of the mist is beginning to clear.

The future may not be cheap

The monks in Kells Abbey probably felt as unhappy about the price of vellum as most librarians feel about journal subscription rates today; certainly their budgets are under as much pressure as ever. There is a perception, however, in the academic and library communities that digital dissemination of science publishing will lower costs of access, these having been borne in preparing the printed version. This overlooks the fact that publishers have spent very large sums installing systems so that text can be retrieved in both print and digital formats. Equally, as journals move to simultaneous digital and print publication, only the costs of paper and posting will be saved.

Most companies and institutions now have a website and much of the content on the Web is little more than promotional information. However, valuable scientific information is usually accessible only after some kind of payment by the user or is available free as a service from the institution, perhaps under some commercial sponsorship. Science publishing now includes video, audio, still image, and interactive data in its digital formats and processing these extra media will need to be paid for. These additional media are becoming integral to publication; they are no longer "bells and whistles" and they are expensive to process.

Libraries will probably continue to buy access to digital information via intermediaries rather than directly from the publisher's server, though they will probably form geographical or special interest consortia to do so. They will pay annual subscriptions to regularly used publications; less frequently accessed titles will be paid for on a "transactional" basis.

Outside the library, individuals will eventually have to pay for access to their required information, as part of a membership fee for their relevant society or association, as a direct subscription to the publisher who will provide an access password, or by way of a transactional access fee for material they use only infrequently.

How it might work

Only Web enthusiasts imagine that science will no longer be published on paper, but only on the Internet. Apart from the unpleasantness of spending any length of time reading a cathode ray tube and the simple pleasure and convenience of holding and reading from a well printed book or journal, the history of technical innovation over the past 50 years indicates that new technologies may change those that came before but they rarely destroy them. There are more radio stations than there were before the introduction of television; far from video killing the cinema, the Hollywood studios are busier than ever and property developers pay handsomely to build multiscreen cinema complexes. We may very well end up with more printed journals, rather than less, published for special interest groups within the larger specialty subject, with the "complete" journal being accessed in libraries, either in traditional printed form or, more likely, in digital format.

Archiving science books and journals is a major challenge. It is likely that the bits and bytes which make up the archive of a journal or scientific book will not be stored on either the publisher's or the library's server. We are seeing the emergence of digital warehouses, to which publishers are delivering the digital version of their books and journals and from which librarians and individuals are accessing them. The computing and telecommunications technologies are all in place to make it very simple. The national libraries might well become the ultimate archive, providing permanent access to digitally formatted science information.

Most publishers will have their own Web servers; on these will be placed all the promotional and bibliographical information relating to their publications, including searchable tables of contents and full structured abstracts, prior to and after publication. These abstracts and tables of contents will contain hypertext links to the full text of the article stored in the digital warehouses such as BIDS (Bath University), OCLC in Ohio, or HighWire Press in California. Publishers might well also post current articles and book chapters on their own website for limited periods, all in full text and without any access charge. The sites will be used for every kind of communication with the publisher, journal editors, and authors, including peer review.

CD-ROMs will continue to perform two key functions: to provide archives of individual and sometimes collected journal titles, mainly for use by personal subscribers rather than libraries. They will also be used as a delivery "platform" for updating information stored on the hard disk of the user's PC.

It should be fun

The Internet has caught everyone's attention. Since the emergence of the World Wide Web, computers have stopped computing and started connecting. For the scientists and researchers, the ability to move words and, more significantly, data around cheaply and easily is a qualitative change to what happened before: a true paradigm shift, just like the invention of movable type. Before the Internet, computers were for the initiated; among authors and scientists, communication is now virtually impossible without them.

Some even wonder whether direct communication between special interest groups of science on the Internet will replace learned societies and their journals. The general consensus among most disciplines seems to be that there remains a need for some kind of peer review process, with all its deficiencies. Endorsement by an established and widely recognised body or publication is likely to remain. The extent to which the Internet is used by researchers and editors before "publication" is likely to vary from subject to subject and will depend largely on the degree of security required.

One thing the Internet can do that is impossible in the print medium is to establish the "dynamic" journal. Grouping a paper with its follow up correspondence and comments drawn from different issues of a journal and perhaps even from different journal titles into a single source on the Web is a major breakthrough, universally welcomed by the scientific community. Publishers and librarians are currently developing linking technologies to improve this process.

Publishers can now alert readers and researchers by email about new articles, letters, and other information that will be of interest to them. There is some evidence that not all readers are wholly in favour of this, usually because they do not have the time to read all the articles about which they are notified. In general, however, using the Internet as a two way communication medium is precisely what makes it so very different from anything that has gone before.

What next?

Over the next five years, more and more communication between authors, referees, publishers, and readers will be conducted over the Net. As authors, research institutions, and publishers resolve the complex questions of copyright, we can look forward to wide access to scientific information that earlier generations could not have imagined. We face a banquet of options that is hard to digest. But there are some signposts as to what the future will look like. The cheap will displace the expensive, digital technology will sit alongside print, and the simple to use will displace the complex. Marketing people and technicians are key members in any digital development team; pride of place, however, must go to the behavioural psychologist.

Could another revolution like the Internet storm the world of science communication again within the next few years, the "future" envisaged in the title of this chapter? It will certainly be improved in that time and as domestic television switches to digital technology, access to the Internet might become virtually universal in the developed world. Software will become at once more elaborate and simple to use, and it will become easier and easier to move large amounts of information around. It is hard to conceive, though, that we will see again in our lifetime anything as truly revolutionary as the Internet.

Index

Page numbers printed in *italic* refer to boxes